This is the second of three discussions concerned with psychosocial and cultural aspects of patient care in general hospitals. Each discussion deals with a different topic, none of which has received systematic examination by most hospitals of this kind. Hence, it was decided to publish these papers separately as small monographs under the generic title *Newer Dimensions of Patient Care*. The first paper, published in 1961, dealt with the planned use of the physical and social environment of the hospital for therapeutic purposes. The third, tentatively scheduled to appear in 1963, will present facts and concepts drawn primarily from sociological and anthropological literature to supplement current psychological knowledge about persons in the role of patients.

Newer Dimensions of
PATIENT CARE

Part 2   Improving Staff Motivation and
Competence in the General Hospital

Esther Lucile Brown, Ph.D.

RUSSELL SAGE FOUNDATION

NEW YORK • 1962

"He's a man, not a bureaucrat.
And I'm a man, not a bureaucrat.
But add us all up and we're a bureaucracy."

Quoted from John Medelman's
"It's Been a Long Snow" in
Harper's Magazine, September, 1960.

CONTENTS

INTRODUCTION

IN THE FIRST OF THIS SERIES of monographs on patient care in general hospitals an attempt was made to picture the anxiety, frustration, boredom, and loneliness that are concomitants of hospitalization for many patients.[1] Perhaps the most frequent criticism of the hospital is its coldness and impersonal atmosphere, with its lack of consideration for the patient as an individual human being. Various relatively simple changes in the use of the physical and social environment of the hospital were suggested as possible means for alleviating some of the boredom and sense of aloneness, and for reducing the sharp difference between the furnishings and atmosphere of the institution and those of the home to which patients are accustomed.

Like its predecessor, this monograph is also concerned with how patient care can be improved. The focus of attention shifts, however, from the physical and social environment as instrumentalities to the hospital staffs that provide direct patient care. Because of their preponderant numbers and their close proximity to patients, particular attention will be given to the nursing staff. Sometimes hospital personnel will be seen in interaction with patients; frequently, however, they will be viewed in their relationships with the members of their work groups. Because we assume that the formal organization and the social system of a hospital are important determinants of what staff think, how they feel, and what they do, much attention will be devoted to organizational and operational arrangements, particularly on the patient floors.

[1] *Newer Dimensions of Patient Care.* Part 1: The Use of the Physical and Social Environment of the General Hospital for Therapeutic Purposes. Russell Sage Foundation, New York, 1961.

From these various examinations it is hoped to gain more comprehensive and deeper understanding of the reasons that care is considered painfully inadequate by many persons experiencing it. The examinations, moreover, will lay a base for judging the possible usefulness of suggestions, drawn from social science literature and experimental efforts in many places, that seek to offer some partial solutions to the problems encountered.

SHORTAGE OF PERSONNEL

Before we can begin to look at the roles of staff and their effectiveness within the hospital setting, some brief reference must be made to the "burning question" of shortage of personnel. Shortages are the most frequent and sometimes almost the only reason given, except financial stringencies, for inadequacies in patient care. Across the length and breadth of the United States hospitals continuously deplore the fact that they cannot provide more individualized attention because of their numerical limitations in staff. The unparalleled expansion in hospital and other health services since World War II, the growing complexity of medicine, and the length and expense of professional training contribute to these shortages.

Since nurses constitute the largest group among the health professions and since they are indispensable to the running of hospitals and providing direct patient care, "the shortage of nurses" has received urgent and often vociferous attention from hospital administrators, doctors, and the public. So much frustration has accompanied the failure to recruit nurses for hospital positions, to say nothing of community nursing, that the uninformed listener might readily conclude that their number was decreasing. Instead, it is increasing both in actual figures and in proportion to population. For many hospitals, moreover, the basic problem is not the recruitment of sufficient nurses numerically. It is the rapid turnover of staff nurses that keeps recruiting a continuous process, and the difficulty of finding persons with the desired qualifications of professional education, experience, and personality to fill important supervisory, administrative, and teaching positions.

More recently and quietly word has begun to be widespread that physicians are too few the country over, and are increasing too slowly to keep pace with growth in population, while some of the specialties like psychiatry need to be enlarged many fold to meet the demand for service. Because a long list of technical procedures that were formerly carried out by doctors has been handed over in whole or in part to nurses, shortage of physicians in general hospitals did not become so quickly or so readily apparent as it would have otherwise. This transferring of responsibility for medical procedures has contributed to the nursing shortage, without solving the problem of numerical insufficiency of doctors.

The utilization of many foreign physicians as house staff has also served to alleviate some of the immediate and crucial difficulties. Since the large majority of these doctors are in the United States only for brief periods of supposed postgraduate training, they offer no solution to the overall problem of quantitative adequacy. It is now finally recognized by the professional associations in medicine, the federal and state governments, and the educated laity that the situation may become progressively worse unless additional medical schools are opened and the enrollment in some of the existing schools is increased, or there is further reallocation of medical duties on a more clearly recognized and systematic basis.

If the number of nurses and physicians falls far below what could profitably be used, the picture is much more dismal in those newer professions for which recruitment and training facilities are exceedingly limited. Medical and psychiatric social workers, physical and occupational or recreational therapists, dietitians, dentists, and various kinds of highly skilled laboratory technicians are progressively regarded as essential members of the staffs of general hospitals, while clinical psychologists and other behavioral scientists are beginning to be employed in more than psychiatric institutions. Except for the most favored hospitals, recruitment of any considerable number of these health workers presents real difficulty.

"SHORTAGES" AS A RATIONALIZATION

Shortages of every category of personnel certainly exist in varying degrees. However, they are only one reason for inadequacies in staff care of patients and may be relatively less impor tant, except in large institutions for the mentally ill and other long-term patients, than they have been made to appear. Short- ages are generally least apparent in teaching hospitals associated with medical schools, and in medical and surgical hospitals oper- ated by the Veterans Administration; many of the voluntary hospitals in some parts of the United States are even overstaffed when compared with national averages or with their European counterparts.

In its statewide nursing surveys the Division of Nursing Re- sources of the United States Public Health Service found hospi- tals, for example, where the average number of hours of nursing care available per patient was one and one-half times as much as recommended practice, and more than twice as much as compar- able hospitals in the area provided to patients.[1] Yet in these supposedly favored institutions one also hears unending com- plaints of too few people to permit more individualized attention to patients. The extensive research program of some hospitals, as well as the education of medical and nursing students, interns, and residents often demands an appreciably enlarged nursing staff.[2] In many instances, however, one is led to conclude that the term "shortages" refers not merely to numerical insufficiencies and to problems such as finding the right person for a particular position. It may also be used as a rationalization to cover short- comings in hospital performance that have not been carefully defined and analyzed.[3]

When *Change and Dilemma in the Nursing Profession* was pub- lished in 1957, Virginia H. Walker noted in her chapter, "Obser-

[1] Abdellah, Faye G., and Eugene Levine, *Effect of Nurse Staffing on Satisfaction with Nursing Care.* American Hospital Association, Monograph Series, no. 4, Chicago, 1958, p. 1.

[2] A memorandum prepared for the writer by Richard Elwell, staff member of the Department of Medicine and Surgery, Veterans Administration Central Office, sug- gests that "an interesting phenomenon comparable to Parkinson's Law is at work. As more personnel—whether nursing, medical, or associated clinical services— are added to the staff and find their way to the ward, an increasing number of nurs- ing personnel are required to attend to staff needs rather than to patient needs. Problems related to the interactions between staff appear to multiply, and the attention of more and more persons is diverted to staff interpersonal relationships rather than staff-patient relationships."

[3] Levine, Eugene, "Nurse Staffing in Hospitals," *American Journal of Nursing,* vol. 61, September, 1961, pp. 65–68.

vations on the Nursing Service," that the majority of nurses interviewed in the hospital under study stated that they wanted to feel assured that the patients for whom they were responsible had good care. However, there was evidence that when these nurses were given an opportunity to establish the desired interpersonal relationships with the patients, they made little observable effort to do it. "This," Miss Walker concluded, "is one of the major dilemmas in the profession today."[1]

Some of the nurses who read the book may recall their reluctance to accept Miss Walker's statement as applicable to other than the particular hospital described. But two recently published reports of nursing care buttress her conclusion. They suggest that something was clearly wrong in each of the hospitals studied, and what was wrong was not solved by the introduction of more graduate nurses.

The School of Nursing of the State University of Iowa decided to test the widely held assumption that a patient's welfare is directly related to the amount and quality of nursing care he receives.[2] If the size of a ward nursing staff were increased without increasing the patient load, according to the hypothesis stated, the staff would automatically redistribute their time in such a way that more time would be allocated to those nursing activities that would be of most benefit to the patients. The results of the experiments did not support this hypothesis. Some of the additional staff time was spent in direct patient care, to be sure, but a large proportion was spent in personal activities. The increase in time devoted to direct patient care, moreover, produced no appreciable increase in the average level of patient welfare.

An in-service educational program was then introduced, supposedly to help these particular nurses improve the quality of patient care. The subsequent experiments showed no improvement in patient welfare resulting from this program, although nursing care may have been improved, and none resulting from combined staff increases and in-service education.

[1] Reissman, Leonard, and John H. Rohrer, editors, *Change and Dilemma in the Nursing Profession.* J. P. Putnam's Sons, New York, 1957, p. 43.

[2] The Nurse Utilization Project Staff of the State University of Iowa, *An Investigation of the Relation Between Nursing Activity and Patient Welfare* published by the State University, Iowa City, 1960. See "Introduction" and "Summary and Conclusions" for results of the experiments.

One of the conclusions reached by the study was that the point beyond which increases in staffing are impractical was much closer to levels existing in the hospital under consideration than had formerly been thought true. Much the same conclusion was reached from experiments in staffing patterns on two units of each of two hospitals in Kansas City.[1] Changes were made in the ratio of staff nurses to auxiliary personnel and in the ratio of all personnel to patients, in an effort to discover whether "an optimum number of hours of nursing care" could be determined. The study team had expected that when more staff nurses were introduced they would spend a greater amount of time with patients. Although some nurses did spend more time, most of them chose to do other things.

Perhaps the most unexpected result of the study was the nurses' reactions on the floor that had been heavily staffed in proportion to the number of patients and also of nursing aides. These nurses complained of boredom, restlessness, and feeling tired. According to their perception "there was just so much work to be done, and after this was accomplished the task was finished."[2] The authors of the report commented that work appeared "to be defined in blocks (or areas) of discrete segments rather than as a continuous flow of events in relation to a central issue (in this case, the patient). By viewing work as segments, the patient is relegated to a secondary position. As a result nursing tasks are separated from the patient, in the nurse's eyes." The authors concluded their interpretation with the perceptive statement that the regulator of tasks for many nurses is not the needs of the patient but "time"—the proper time to give medications and treatments, to see that the patient has his bath and the bed is made up, to take a "coffee break."

THE FUNCTIONAL METHOD OF PATIENT CARE

From these studies some of the causes of poor patient care besides shortages begin to become apparent. The method of functional, rather than case, assignment is unquestionably a stum-

[1] New, Peter Kong-ming, Gladys Nite, and Josephine M. Callahan, *Nursing Service and Patient Care: A Staffing Experiment.* Community Studies, Inc., Kansas City, Publication 119, November, 1959, pp. 73ff.

[2] *Ibid.,* p. 75.

bling block. When nurses are assigned specific tasks, such as administering medications to all patients in the unit or performing highly technical procedures wherever needed, and are not given responsibility for the comprehensive nursing care of any patients, it is not surprising that they take little interest in patients as persons. Almost inevitably, they will be procedure-centered rather than patient-centered.

One should not assume that such lack of interest is limited to nurses. Because the nursing profession has sponsored or engaged in many studies during the past decade of nurses and nursing. data about its problems are often more readily available than they are for the other professions. Anyone, however, who has had an opportunity to watch medical and surgical house staff at work is aware that the problems are much the same in medicine as in nursing. Young men, who are frequently hurried, overworked, and perhaps anxious, enter patients' rooms to take case histories, make physical examinations, or give treatments. Frequently they forget even to introduce themselves. Many hospitals have sought to remedy such an oversight by providing nameplates for all categories of staff to wear. Thus, if a patient can see the plate or is experienced enough to differentiate between the various types of uniform worn, he is able to tell whether his busy and seemingly distracted visitor is a young physician or a laboratory technician.

The desire to communicate with the patient and to develop sound interpersonal relations appears to be regarded by house staffs "as a luxury not expected in nonprivate practice."[1] That these physicians realize lack of individual attention will not be conducive to their attracting private patients is borne out by the remark one occasionally hears a resident make when he is about to open his office. "Now I will have to begin to pay attention to interpersonal relations," says he. The listener is inclined to inquire how well prepared he will be for such an important but delicate undertaking after years of treating patients primarily as if they were objects.

A clinical professor in a university hospital, who seeks more individualized care for his patients and is also interested in staff

---

[1] Brant, Charles S., Herbert Volk, and Bernard Kutner, "Psychological Preparation for Surgery," *Public Health Reports*, vol. 73, November, 1958, p. 1005.

development, makes a practice of telephoning to the appropriate intern before the patient is admitted to the hospital. In considerable detail the intern is told who the patient is, what he does, what he is like as a person. Thus the attending physician hopes that the young doctor will feel that he is not suddenly encountering a total stranger, and that he will be able to do something more while taking a case history than to ask a great many questions in a perfunctory manner.

Hopefully, physical and occupational therapists and social workers are in somewhat less harried positions and hence give relatively more individualized attention to patients. Certainly, other observers besides the writer have commented on the warmth, friendly atmosphere, and decreased tension that seemed to characterize many of the physical and occupational units they have seen. Some of these units, however, are extremely busy and even the scheduling of all the patients referred is difficult and tension-producing.

Physical and occupational therapists and social workers work primarily with patients referred to them by physicians and often on the basis of fairly specific orders about what should be done. For some of them who are function-centered rather than patient-centered, concern does not extend beyond the carrying out of the doctor's order. But many, and particularly social workers trained in working with patients through a carefully established relationship, complain because of the limitations imposed on them. Often they hear of patients who, in their estimation, would benefit greatly from their services but are not referred, or patients who are referred for therapeutic intervention that they consider much too restricted in scope.

Social workers, for example, may conclude that painstaking psychological preparation of a particular patient is indicated if he is to be able to accept drastic change in physical condition and way of life; yet they may be requested to make quick assessment of the environmental situation and suggest a plan for new living arrangements. Frequently, representatives of all these groups feel that the medical profession does not know how to use their skills adequately, and pays little attention to them. When these feelings are strong enough, such persons can perhaps scarcely keep from transmitting their frustrations to patients.

CONSEQUENCES OF THE FUNCTIONAL METHOD

Clearly a concomitant of the functional method of giving patient care has been the division of work among a rapidly increasing number and variety of persons. At the turn of the century doctors and nurses and their students ran hospitals and cared for patients with the assistance of a few persons in the kitchen, laundry, boiler room, and an occasional office. Today a therapeutic team may consist of several medical and nursing specialists and representatives of a half-dozen other professional or technically trained groups, besides several auxiliary helpers. In addition, the hospital has become an elaborate organization of many departments operated under the general supervision of a hospital administrator and his assistants.

What has been happening in the overall growth and complexity of institutions caring for the sick has naturally had its counterpart on the patient floors. In an attempt to use physicians and nurses at something approaching the highest level of their competence, many medical functions have been transferred, not only to nurses as already mentioned but to laboratory technicians, dietitians, physical and occupational therapists, social workers, and sometimes chaplains. Scores of functions formerly performed by nurses or nursing students have been allocated to practical nurses, aides, ward secretaries, maids, cleaning men, persons who transport food trays, and so on. To plan for the distribution of tasks among such a variety of persons is no easy undertaking. To keep the resulting system running with any considerable efficiency requires extensive and competent supervision.

Even at best such a system creates many problems both for staff and for patients. Work becomes so subdivided that many of the tasks, performed by persons in the lower echelons, are highly repetitive and the prestige attached to them is low. Hence the work tends to be viewed as limited in interest. Monotony and low prestige are likely to produce decreasing motivation, which in turn fosters job turnover, or frequent absences.[1] And what is perhaps more important, low motivation fosters a tendency in the employee to get through the workday as comfortably as possi-

[1] Melbin, Murray, "Organization Practice and Individual Behavior: Absenteeism Among Psychiatric Aides," *American Sociological Review*, vol. 26, February, 1961, pp. 14–23.

ble; coffee breaks, chit-chat with the members of one's work group, or simply standing around, are often substituted for meeting patients' requests promptly, cheerfully, and without the appearance of being hurried.

Administrators and supervisors are well aware that severe problems have been created by the subdivision of labor, and that their particular hospital has not escaped its share. But, interestingly, they often seem unaware of what occurs in various parts of their institution at the point of direct patient care. Most of the time of administrators is spent elsewhere than on the patient floors. Generally, moreover, they have not been trained to make situational observations, and when they visit a floor it is usually for a specific purpose. They have not had the experience of one physician who, when he was unexpectedly made assistant superintendent of a psychiatric hospital, learned much about the institution and his job by sitting for an hour every morning for a year on the various wards.

One of the reasons physicians and supervisory nurses do not know more about what actually happens is that their white uniforms and their positions of authority within the hierarchical structure of the hospital put them at a disadvantage in making observations. The supervisor of the private pavilion in a large voluntary hospital once remarked that she considered nurses excellent actors, capable of changing behavior and rearranging the environment rapidly if they knew she was coming to their floor. She concluded that she had no opportunity to see typical conditions unless she succeeded in getting to a unit quite unexpectedly. Thanks to the efficiency of the "grapevine" or other warning signal, ward staff are frequently alerted to the imminent arrival of a doctor or supervisory nurse. By the time such a person reaches the floor they are busily at work.

The following example will illustrate the kind of behavior that a visitor in street clothes may see more readily than a supervisory nurse. It is presented in order to suggest how neglectful ward staff can be of virtually helpless patients, not because they want or intend to be neglectful but rather because their motivation is low. They work, if our interpretation be correct, where they receive too little praise, encouragement, and psychological support;

where the hospital seems uninterested in them personally; and where the condition of the patients is often hard to tolerate and perhaps anxiety-inducing. Lest the reader conclude that this example is unrepresentative, we must note that other situations observed in hospitals for acute sickness could have been substituted. The social factors involved were, in fact, so similar that it was hard to choose one illustration for presentation here.

Frequently on Sunday afternoons the writer visited a friend suffering from advanced multiple sclerosis, who was hospitalized on a men's neurological unit of a well-known hospital for long-term patients. This unit was composed of an open ward with fifteen beds, and of rooms for one or two patients accommodating about an equal number of persons. There was no system of lights, bells, or other communication with the nurse's station, and that station was located in an office from which almost no part of the unit was visible. Most of the patients, furthermore, were in a badly regressed condition.

The writer would sometimes sit for twenty-five minutes without a single staff member's coming into the ward, even to see if the patients were all right. When she could stand the situation no longer, she would tell her friend that she was going to get a drink of water or find ice cream for him. Out of sight, just around the corner of the unit, she would discover perhaps six men aides smoking cigarettes, joking, and laughing. In the nursing office with the door closed was a practical nurse who was the charge nurse of the unit.

According to the report of her friend, the practical nurse on one of the three shifts was able to supervise the aides efficiently. The patients were certain they knew the moment she entered the unit, even though they could not see her. The aides were immediately busy and during her tour of duty they were available and helpful. This practical nurse also spent much of her time giving medications and treatments and "keeping things going" as best she could. On the other two shifts the women practical nurses were apparently too inexperienced and psychologically too insecure to supervise several Negro and Puerto Rican men aides. They retreated to the office, closed the door, and stayed there as much as possible. "Goofing off" by the aides was said to be frequent.

Medical care was provided the patients almost exclusively by residents, who served the neurological unit for only three months before being replaced by other residents. The period was scarcely long enough for patients, staff, and doctors to become acquainted with each other and hopefully to settle into some kind of mutually supporting routine. Then the residents were gone, perhaps without even mentioning the fact that they were being transferred. If a patient had established a strong relationship with one of these doctors, as had the man with multiple sclerosis, he felt suddenly lost with no one to whom to turn.

Because most of these patients were considered past the stage where rehabilitation would benefit them, they received little attention from senior physicians or from physical and occupational therapists. Usually the few social workers were more needed elsewhere. When a nursing supervisor made her occasional tour, it may be assumed that word of her arrival generally preceded her and she found everything "under control." Two of the three practical nurses and the aides had good reasons for not wanting to report about each other to her.

At a subsequent time members of the administrative staff of this hospital and the writer were discussing possible experimental projects, based on social science concepts and methods of evaluation, that might be introduced to see if ward patient care could be improved generally. The writer inquired whether a project might not well be initiated in a part of the hospital where the patient care was most inadequate. One of the administrators mentioned both the neurological and cancer units as unsatisfactory. A careful explanation was made of the fact that it was impossible to obtain graduate nurses to be head nurses of those units, not only because of the discouraging nature of the diseases but also because of the drabness and nonfunctional construction of the buildings.

Reference was also made to the fact that since almost all patient care had to be provided by aides, the units were more generously staffed than would have been true had graduate or even practical nurses been available. The hospital obviously hoped that by supplying more "hands and feet" patients would receive more care. It probably did not know that studies were beginning to appear that seemed to indicate that, beyond a certain point, additional staff are likely to spend much time interacting with staff rather than with patients.

The administrators stated that the outmoded units were to be rebuilt almost immediately. That step, plus others that were being taken to attract nurses to the hospital as a whole, might accomplish much in helping to solve the staffing problem on those particular units. Short of better staff and better supervision, the administration did not see what it could do. It was the same dilemma in which countless other hospitals have found themselves!

Honest, sincere persons assumed that they knew the nature of the problem with which they were faced and were trying to find a solution. It seemed to the writer, however, that they were unaware of the degree of seriousness of the problem: the fact that not even safe nursing care was being guaranteed patients on the neurological unit. Had the persons in that conference room been able to observe the unit at length and unrecognized, we believe that some concerted effort would have been made immediately to bring about change, even though the services of graduate nurses could not be obtained. We think it likely that the administration would have been willing to embark on a social science experiment, such as had been tried with considerable success in psychiatric hospitals, designed to raise the motivation and competence of the aides and two of the three practical nurses who staffed the unit. We believe, furthermore, that once word about an ongoing experiment had spread through the institution, it would have attracted the interest of graduate nurses.

BETTER UTILIZATION OF HUMAN RESOURCES

The director of a relatively very good but large general hospital once remarked that his institution had been provided with almost lavish facilities and with an amazingly generous supply of professionally trained persons of all kinds. The problem, said he, was how the hospital could learn to use its human resources as well as it had learned to use diagnostic procedures and treatment facilities, including complex machines.

In that statement he probably spoke for every hospital of any appreciable size that believes it should attempt to serve patients as persons. The present system of subdivision of labor that begins to resemble the assembly line of an industrial plant appears to yield satisfaction neither for many of the staff nor for a considerable proportion of the patients. It has also failed to yield the degree of hoped-for efficiency. Whether greater perfection of the present system of organization and operation would produce noticeable amelioration of current conditions is doubtful.[1] Some hospitals take pride in the skilled attention they have given to the development of administrative rules and procedures to meet every exigency they could envisage. Yet those very hospitals may be as lacking in the communication and coordination necessary to get a missing fork delivered to a patient before his meal is cold, or to get a slipped oxygen mask replaced before the patient de-

[1] For a pertinent discussion of questionable trends in industry, see the section "Tighter Management Controls and Their Impact Upon the Employees" in Chris Argyris' *Personality and Organization:* The Conflict Between System and the Individual, Harper and Bros., New York, 1957, pp. 130ff.

velops serious apprehension, as hospitals that have no such proficiency in their administrative offices.

Social scientists interested in experimental undertakings in industry have begun to question the wisdom of drawing charts of organizational structure and formulating plans and directives for operation without giving equal attention to how employees are likely to react to the social system created. It was long assumed that if management attempted to meet workers' demands for wages and benefits, employees could and would be expected to fit into the existing organizational pattern. Even though interchangeability of persons was required for many of the jobs, it was almost taken for granted that the "fit" between employee and organization would be generally good. In the light of knowledge developed by the behavioral sciences and applied in recent studies of industry, that assumption appears naive and the probable results unfortunate, unless by chance the requirements of the organization should be congruent with the psychological and social needs of the workers.

If such an assumption may have unfortunate consequences for industry, the effects could be scarcely short of disastrous for hospitals where the object of the average worker's task is a human being. The basic question, therefore, becomes one of attempting to see whether the psychosocial, as well as the economic, needs of staff and the objectives of the institution can be harmonized sufficiently to foster better utilization of the hospital's human resources.

In the chapters that follow, definition of the needs of staff will receive first consideration. It will be taken for granted that unless such needs can be reasonably well met, the staff will resort to a wide variety of conscious and unconscious means for not meeting patients' needs. An attempt will then be made to look at the organizational structure and the formal social system of the hospital to see how their requirements conform to those of the staff. Wherever possible, descriptions of practices and experimental undertakings will be included that seem to offer some promise of making the "fit" between staff and institution more comfortable, and hence of encouraging personnel to use themselves more whole-heartedly in caring for patients.

Chapter 1

PSYCHOLOGICAL AND SOCIAL NEEDS
OF STAFF

A RECENTLY PUBLISHED BOOK, *Personnel: The Human Problems of Management*, emphasizes by its very title the current focus of attention of many writers who are interesting themselves in how management and labor can work together more effectively.[1] In the rapidly growing literature consideration is increasingly devoted to the psychosocial needs of employees, as predicated on the basis of social science theory and an expanding body of experimental studies. Regardless of differences in the particular behavioral concepts selected for major attention, there is general consensus that more than the economic needs of personnel must receive careful notice from management if an organization is to be able to meet its chief objectives over any appreciable period of time.

This literature is in sharp contrast to the earlier writing of Frederick W. Taylor, father of the "Taylor system" of scientific management, and his disciples who greatly influenced industrial development. Taylor was interested in how workers might perform specific acts most efficiently; he gave little attention to aspects of human personality. He advocated that every job should be kept as simple as possible, with the number of separate operations reduced to the minimum. "Each man," he wrote, "must learn how to give up his own particular way of doing things, adapt his methods to the many new standards, and grow accustomed to receiving and obeying directions covering details, large and small, which in the past have been left to his individual

[1] Strauss, George, and Leonard R. Sayles, *Personnel: The Human Problems of Management.* Prentice-Hall, Inc., Englewood Cliffs, N. J., 1960.

19

judgment."[1] Taylor himself became aware that specialization through division of labor might eventually kill opportunity for the worker to show ingenuity or creativity.[2]

The attitude of many behavioral scientists to the Taylor system is perhaps well summarized by the following quotation:

> Scientific management has failed to utilize properly the greatest resource at its command: the complex and multiple capacities of people. On the contrary . . . it has deliberately sought to utilize as narrow a band of personality and as narrow a range of ability as ingenuity could devise. The process has been fantastically wasteful for industry and society.[3]

THE BEHAVIORAL REQUIREMENTS OF PERSONNEL

Let us now turn to some of the aspects of human personality that scientific management supposedly neglected, to the loss of industry and society. Since attention can be given only to a limited number, those selected for emphasis may differ slightly from those that other writers would choose. Even the terminology used in describing them and the exact meaning behind the terminology will differ somewhat from writer to writer. Readers will undoubtedly be in general agreement, however, that these personality needs are clearly recognizable, vital, and shared in varying degrees by almost everyone.

1. Social Approval

Throughout the entire life span most persons crave social approval, whether they are aware of that fact or not. The desire to win it—or to win social status, in the language of the sociologists —is a strong motivating force. In the hope of achieving social

---

[1] *Shop Management.* Harper and Bros., New York, 1919, p. 113.

[2] As illustration of what ingenuity and creativity have accomplished in recent decades when there was opportunity for them to be applied to the solution of some of the great agricultural, industrial, and mining problems of America, see Ira Wolfert's fascinating saga, *An Epidemic of Genius,* Simon and Schuster, Inc., New York, 1960. The reader will probably conclude that the day of "miracles" is not past.

[3] Worthy, James C., "Some Observations on Frederick W. Taylor and the Scientific Management Movement." An address presented to the Society of Applied Anthropology, New York, April 19, 1954; quoted in Strauss and Sayles' *Personnel: The Human Problems of Management,* p. 37.

approval some will struggle valiantly to own a fine home, drive a conspicuous automobile, send their children to private schools, or join exclusive clubs. Others see their opportunity to advance in social status through holding political office, being promoted to "more important" positions, making public speeches, or writing technical books for their professional colleagues to read. Still others look for social approval through their highly perfected skills, whether manifested in swimming matches, polo playing, fine handwrought furniture, or obtaining competitive funds for research purposes.

To work is looked on with favor in our culture and hence tends to bestow general social approval on the worker. More importantly, it is only through work for pay that most people can find the wherewithal to buy the symbols of social status or can obtain the necessary opportunity to display skills and talents. As Dr. J. A. C. Brown has commented, "Work is an essential part of a man's life, since it is that aspect of his life which gives him status and binds him to society."[1] Hence it can safely be said, not merely on the basis of logical deduction or general observation, but of research studies made in recent decades, that most persons like to work.

Because management long assumed and sometimes continues to assume that men are by nature lazy and do not want to work, this is a discovery of vital importance. It suggests that if any considerable number of persons in a particular organization, in this instance the hospital, tend to "goof off" whenever possible or otherwise show little interest in their work, an attempt should be made to find the reason. Often it has appeared, as in the instance presented in the Introduction, that such behavior results from the fact that the worker is receiving no praise or other positive form of recognition, or thinks he is receiving none. In essence, the social approval he craves is being denied him.

2. Sense of Accomplishment

Just as most people like social approval, so they also like a sense of accomplishment. This is a second psychosocial requirement to

[1] *The Social Psychology of Industry:* Industry in the Factory. Penguin Books, Inc., Baltimore, 1954, p. 187.

which reference must be made. Here again work provides a primary way for gaining satisfaction through making or doing something, and doing it well. Some men say they like the feeling of being tired at night, if the tiredness comes from a "good day's work." By contrast, work that seems pointless, or does not provide a sense of achievement, leads to frustration. One hears the familiar statement, "The trouble with this work is that I don't have any feeling of accomplishment. I'm just nobody, doing nothing, getting nowhere. I'm just a cog, so small I'd never be missed."[1]

Lack of a sense of accomplishment is by no means limited to persons who are "just nobody." Many an important position has been filled by someone selected on the basis of personality, education, and experience. Yet that person may suffer great frustration because of carrying too much responsibility without the necessary accompanying authority, or having insufficient autonomy to make the changes and develop the programs he considers important or inadequate opportunity to wield the power demanded by a neurotic need to achieve. Two examples of these generalizations will be given from the hospital world.

Those who have listened to nurses talking to each other will recall how frequently they, and particularly the head nurses, complain of being tired, too tired often to do anything constructive in the evening. "I've run all day long and yet I haven't accomplished half what I should have. And worst of all, I've had no time to spend with the patients." Since most of these nurses are young and well, fatigue can probably be attributed to lack of preparation for their jobs or to frustration. These shortcomings may well be significant causes of high turnover. Later, when the social system of the hospital is examined, it will be seen that the nursing service, as a whole, and head nurses, particularly, are in the unenviable position of having too many "bosses" and not having authority commensurate with their responsibility. As a consequence they are frequently robbed of a much needed sense of accomplishment.

One might well assume that persons occupying the top professional and administrative positions in a general hospital would

[1] Strauss and Sayles, *Personnel: The Human Problems of Management*, p. 19.

benefit from a sense of large achievement, if for no other reason than because of the position attained. Interestingly, however, such persons are generally not easy to satisfy. They belong to the group that are highly motivated to get things done, and may be like the administration of one hospital Dr. Argyris characterized as "pushers, prodders, and go-getters."[1] Under such circumstances they often find themselves suffering from impatience and other inner tensions at the expense of a sense of accomplishment. Failure is exceptionally hard for them to accept. "So it is not difficult to see why these executives are always working harder than is necessary, and setting their goals higher than is expected of them. It is especially important for them not to fail."[2]

3. Sense of the Importance of the Job

Another need experienced by most workers is that their job is important. This need is so closely related to that for accomplishment that it would not receive separate attention here did it not stand at the very core of problems faced by hospital staffs on the lower levels.

Importance is determined largely by social values. Hence almost no one feels sure that his own evaluation corresponds with that of his friends, work group, or boss. In order to benefit psychologically, one's judgment of importance must generally be validated by others or by the nature of the social situation.[3] Since large numbers of persons are hired by hospitals on an interchangeable basis with other persons, supposedly to do the routine work, administration often raises the question of how it can honestly attempt to make these persons feel that what they do as individuals is important.

Thus it fails to note that its value judgment of importance and that of workers on the lower echelons may be quite different. To

[1] Argyris, Chris, *Diagnosing Human Relations in Organizations: A Case Study of a Hospital.* Labor and Management Center, Yale University, New Haven, 1956, p. 102.

[2] *Ibid.*

[3] In *Language and Society* (Random House, New York, 1955, p. 22), Joseph Bram has made the cogent statement: "All human beings are aware of being perceived and evaluated by others; they form an idea of how they are viewed by others; they are preoccupied with being viewed favorably; they keep checking on their fluctuating value on the interactional 'stock market'; their own image of their selves is thus largely a socially produced and internalized conception."

an executive the job of running an elevator is likely to seem dull and boring. But the operator whose car is used by distinguished physicians who greet him every morning, or by patients who are being taken to and from surgery on stretchers, may well believe that he is indispensable to the institution. The hospital itself provides a sense of importance to workers who gain satisfaction from serving others or from taking responsibility for those unable to assume responsibility for themselves. Attitudes of some sectors of the community, moreover, reinforce this sense of importance. "To hear our nursing assistants tell their families and friends about what they do," said a director of nursing service, "would make you believe that they run this hospital." The Spanish-American community where these men aides live appears convinced that working in that particular institution is about the best job a man can have.

In-service training for the preparation of nursing aides furnishes an excellent social situation, the psychological significance of which may have been overlooked by hospital directors, for suggesting to the largest category of personnel that their jobs *are* important. The classroom sessions, demonstrations of the best ways to carry out technical procedures, and finally practice on the ward under the supervision of a nurse, reproduce symbols associated with the training of nurses and doctors. Unfortunately, some of the attitudes later encountered by the aides at work may dispel their early impression.

The problem of filling positions on the lower rungs of the hierarchical ladder is one, in Dr. J. A. C. Brown's opinion, that has been created in large measure by administration. The executive who thinks about how he can find persons "who will do the lowly and dirty work . . . is completely forgetting the quite obvious fact that the lowliness and nastiness of a job are subjective estimates, and that what really matters is the prestige of the job, and, even more important, the prestige of the group for which the job is to be done."[1] This conclusion appears patent in hospitals where physicians and nurses must do many exceedingly unpleasant

---

[1] *The Social Psychology of Industry*, p. 149. As an example of current fiction that has as its major thesis the importance of all *productive work* and the assumption that there is no such thing as a "lousy job" but "only lousy men who don't care to do it," see Ayn Rand's *Atlas Shrugged*, Random House, New York, 1957.

things but where the prestige of these two groups is high. One neurologist worked for many years, as he said, "with blood, guts, and faeces," yet he and his research were internationally known.

For those administrators and supervisors who sincerely want to encourage motivation of staff but have been skeptical about how a sense of importance could be given to personnel such as aides, the research of recent years concerning the behavior of small groups may offer helpful suggestions. Persons conducting this research have questioned the effectiveness of large and expensive undertakings, like the printing of beautifully illustrated booklets that some industries have given to each employee. Management has gone on the assumption that once the worker learned the facts about the industry, he would be proud to identify himself with it. The worker, however, may well have concluded that such lavishness could be only for promotional purposes, and he did not intend "to be a sucker."

Small group research, instead, sees in the worker's immediate peer group and in the interest shown by one or two persons in supervisory positions, appropriate sources for the validation of importance that may have true meaning for the employees. In the next chapter we shall return to the subject of the peer group and the vital role that such groups play in most large organizations. Here we wish to comment on the influence of those persons in supervisory positions. Within the context of the hospital ward or floor, they would generally be the head nurse or leader of the nursing team and the physician responsible for the medical care.

If nursing aides have often concluded that they were the "low men on the totem pole," the behavior of their immediate bosses and also of the staff nurses has frequently justified that conclusion. Nurses are now beginning to feel more comfortable with auxiliary personnel than they did fifteen years ago when it became apparent that such personnel would have to be used in increasing numbers. Understandably they resented the fact that even some of their duties could be performed by women and men who had had very brief training. Considerable effort was expended in attempting to convince nurses that they were rarely being robbed of important functions; they were being upgraded. As a consequence it became relatively easy for those who were still resentful to treat the aides as if the latter were hired to do only the unimportant and unpleasant tasks.

Much progress has been made generally by the two groups in settling into working relations that are less frustrating. Some hospitals, particularly those operated by the federal government, have consistently attempted to increase the prestige of their aides. Their efforts have included excellent in-service training offered progressively, perhaps on two or three levels; provision for advancement in responsibility, rank, and salary; and occasional opportunity for all categories of staff to join in informal social gatherings. In such places the aides appear to have responded with increased commitment to their job and sometimes with less turnover and fewer absences.[1]

Elsewhere, some nurses may still treat aides as if the latter were unworthy of being an integral part of the nursing service. Their lack of generosity of spirit shows itself in their surprise when someone suggests that aides be praised for work well done. "Why should praise be given to people who are only doing what they are paid to do?" Particularly revealing of a major problem of human relations in the hospital is the question nurses rarely ask outright but often imply. "Why should aides get praise when we who are in more responsible positions don't get it?"

If auxiliary personnel often receive less validation from nurses of their importance in patient care than they need, they generally receive almost none from physicians in hospitals for acute disease. (In long-term hospitals the situation is likely to be somewhat different, since most of the care, and sometimes the supervision, is provided by aides and practical nurses.) With the exception of orderlies who may assist doctors with urological dressings and treatments, physicians have little direct contact with auxiliary personnel. They rarely know the names of such persons; they pay scant attention to them. Doctors' communication is with the nurses, generally the head nurse or her assistant, and much of it is limited to information and directives written in the order book or on the patient's chart. Thus, most unfortunately, auxiliary

[1] For a more detailed discussion of psychological means for increasing the effective use of auxiliary personnel, see the writer's article "The Nursing Profession and Auxiliary Personnel" in *Aspects of Public Health Nursing*, World Health Organization, Public Health Papers, no. 4, Geneva, 1961, pp. 23–28.

personnel are cut off from identification with the doctor, the father symbol of strength and authority on the ward, and are forced to rely almost exclusively for psychological support upon the "mother," even though she may sometimes be cold and rejecting.

Two small incidents will illustrate more meaningfully than any generalization how crushing to one's personality neglect can be, and how close is the possible relationship between recognition of the worker's worth and what he will attempt to do on the job when not closely supervised.

In a discussion with third-year medical students who were having their first clinical experience, they spoke of their surprise and dismay at the lack of interest and the carelessness shown by the aides in the city hospital to which they had been assigned. When asked whether any of the physicians, including themselves, were acquainted with or gave attention to the aides, they responded in the negative. Suddenly one student said, "Perhaps the attendants' egos are suffering. Ours are. There isn't a single attending [physician] who so much as knows one of our names. If just one doctor would address us as Mr. ———— you don't know what it would do for our morale!"

* * * *

On the diabetic service of another large teaching hospital the resident physician and the writer stood watching two aides spend as much time in making a bed without a patient in it as one person should require to make two or three beds. Patients were greatly in need of attention, and the general atmosphere of the ward was one of drabness, apathy, and an appalling lack of amenities. The resident was discouraged with the depressing conditions. The head nurse, who was temporarily without even a secretary to answer the telephone, and the "medicine nurse," who was a student, could give no attention except in emergencies to the aides or to ward housekeeping. "What *could* be done?" the resident asked.

We talked about the need all of us have to gain a sense of importance through work. Then we posed the question of what might happen were the doctors to indicate an interest in the aides and their duties, were to ask them day after day for their general observations about some patient, and were to show appreciation whenever they demonstrated greater motivation or more ability to observe and report. The writer learned long afterward that the resident found a way out of his own discouragement through seeing the aides respond, to his great surprise, to the attention he gave them. They began to take an interest in the patients and were proud to be asked their opinions.

This leads to the almost trite remark that practically everyone likes to be consulted and given an opportunity to express opinions and make suggestions. The very fact of being consulted validates for many workers the importance of their job. Yet, the behavior of large institutions is so determined by organizational structure and attitudes of exclusiveness stemming from professional education, that only persons who occupy certain positions are likely to feel free, or are encouraged, to express ideas or even report their observations. It is then but a short step to the conclusion that persons on the lower hierarchical levels have no facts or ideas of importance to express. Like many other expectations about how people will act, this negative expectation may easily be fulfilled. Countless members of hospital staffs, who are in exceptional situations for gathering needed data, have not been consulted for so long that when they are finally asked for information they can think of nothing to say. We shall see in the next chapter how much time and effort may have to be expended in helping such staff members develop to the point where they can become true participants in a therapeutic effort.

4. Security

Security is a fourth behavioral need that cannot be overlooked. In the next chapter the subject of security as psychologically experienced will be implicit in much of the discussion of peer groups, since they are a primary medium for providing security. Here attention will be given to other aspects of the subject.

The term is used in the literature of management and labor in various senses. Often it refers to job security or tenure, and as such is viewed as perhaps more significant than either pay or advancement. In studies of what workers want from their job, "steady work" is likely to appear in first or second place while "tenure" of position is important to executives. Without job security large numbers of persons suffer acute uncertainty. The economic depression of the 1930s with its vast unemployment not only caused great hardship, but conditioned many children so adversely that a search for job security has dogged their steps and has sometimes assumed pathological proportions.

The ever-quickening pace of technological development has caused some of the same manifestations. Workers are robbed of dependence upon themselves since their peculiar abilities are no longer necessary, and automation is feared as wiping out entire large groups of workers. Hence the demand for contractual security that has been strong for almost two decades may become even more pervasive. When a man cannot "depend on himself in the way he once could," Mason Haire reminds us, "he must have contractual assurance that he will be taken care of in the future, that if he is sick he will be paid during the period when he can so easily be replaced, and that his unemployment will be underwritten by someone."[1]

Job security is significant for other reasons besides providing assurance of continuity in earning one's living. Many persons who do not need a pay check are seriously disturbed if robbed through disability, being "laid off," or early retirement, of their customary work world that has provided social contacts, vital satisfaction, and perhaps self-fulfillment.

Fortunately, job security has presented few realistic problems for the health professions since the beginning of World War II. Because of the shortage of personnel of almost every kind, many institutions and agencies have even had to retain persons who lack the ability, preparation, experience, or motivation desired. Some individuals, to be sure, suffer general anxiety that becomes focused upon whether their job is secure, but there are few visible indications of any recession in the health field in the near future. Technological progress, moreover, has not had such devastating effects there as in industry and business.

The assumption was long widespread, and still persists in places in spite of many studies to the contrary, that wages or salary represented the form of security of greatest importance to workers. This assumption is reinforced by the frequent demands particularly of unionized labor for pay increases. It is also reinforced by the tendency of management to offer money and a progressively longer list of benefits to labor, as if it were saying, "We will give you all sorts of material rewards if you will please continue

[1] Haire, Mason, *Psychology in Management.* McGraw-Hill Book Co., New York, 1956, p. 33.

to produce in spite of the human difficulties that you will experience while at work."[1]

For persons on the economic periphery, wages as well as job security are unquestionably of major importance. Money continues to play a considerable role even after financial stringencies have lessened, but in large part because of quite different reasons. If new personnel are paid high salaries to attract their services, persons who have spent years in the organization will insist upon an equal amount. In fact, equity of salary may loom more important than amount among persons on the supervisory levels.[2] Many individuals conceive of their pay check and the luxuries it buys as the visible evidence of success or power when the money in itself has little meaning for them. Some would even be willing to take a decrease in salary, should it appear necessary, provided everyone else was reduced proportionately.

When research workers have asked employees in stable industries to indicate the order of importance to them of a list of items that are supposedly desired by workers, financial remuneration has often been well toward the bottom of their assessment. Some years ago a social scientist discovered, as he organized his interview data on what nurses in a particular hospital wanted, that salary increases across the board took eighth or ninth place among ten items. Salary was mentioned in fourth place, but only in the form of some small readjustment of evening or night schedules. First and second places were given to the nurses' desire that they be blamed less when the fault lay in the social system of the hospital, and that they be praised more often when they did something well!

It is surprising to many persons that hospital staffs have not made more frequent and vigorous demands for higher pay and improved benefits. These persons view institutional salary schedules for almost everyone, except possibly top executives, as very low. Medical house staff and personnel on the aide and maintenance levels often have to depend on their spouses to supplement the family income. Salaries of staff nurses are rarely better than

[1] Argyris, Chris, *Personality and Organization:* The Conflict Between System and the Individual. Harper and Bros., New York, 1957, p. 110.

[2] Herzberg, Frederick, Bernard Mausner, and Barbara Bloch Snyderman, *The Motivation to Work.* John Wiley and Sons, New York, 1959, pp. 116–117.

those of secretaries who are employed from nine until five o'clock in generally pleasant surroundings.

Thanks to a long tradition of the hospital as a charitable enterprise where one works primarily to serve and not for money, and thanks also to the success of these institutions in forestalling or delaying unionization, hospitals have not contemplated offering the material rewards that Argyris points to in industry. Almost every salary increase or fringe benefit has been granted with great reluctance. Nurses have succeeded since World War II in obtaining several modest increases in salary. Recently ward aides, food service and maintenance employees, and even medical house staff have begun to present their case to the public through newspaper advertisements, noon-hour picketing, or other methods exceedingly embarrassing to the hospitals under attack. Hence it is not yet possible to foresee what relative place the pay envelope may assume among hospital personnel.

5. Support in Anxiety-Inducing Situations

Before bringing this section to a close some attention must be given to a very different aspect of security. It is one that receives little attention in the general literature of management and labor but is of the utmost importance in connection with hospitals. We refer to psychological security necessitated by the nature of the work situation. Because of its very function the hospital is an anxiety-inducing institution, a fact of which the laity is generally well aware. Through a long process of conditioning, including (we believe) a great deal of repression and suppression, staff appear to come to terms to an amazing degree with this characteristic of the hospital. They may even come to terms with it to such an extent that some express initial surprise when the hospital is referred to as anxiety-inducing.

However, many cues suggest that situations that might produce anxiety in the individual therapist are often unconsciously avoided, perhaps to the detriment of patients and their families. In Part I of *Newer Dimensions of Patient Care* reference was made to the avoidance of the word "death," regardless of the fact that the hospital knows it must expect death as a frequent visitor. In her account of her husband's death from cancer, Mrs. Werten-

baker notes, "Maybe the 'croakers' and 'stiffs' of medical neo-
phytes are as much fearful euphemisms as 'pass on' and 'gone to
reward on high.'"[1] Considerable sections of her book illustrate
the difficulty that physicians and nurses have in telling a patient
he cannot live, in facing him comfortably if he accepts death
naturally, and in letting him die if incurable.

Anyone who walks hospital floors and listens to staff conversa-
tions is likely to become aware of how little support many physicians and nurses are able to give persons who are designated as
"terminal cases" or as "doing poorly"; how members of the
family are often avoided; and how the calling of a chaplain frequently seems to relieve the staff of a feeling of further responsibility. Unless a patient has a personal physician, the psychological
support he and his family receive may be minimal. This kind of
behavior would seem to result in large part from anxiety produced by a situation with which many persons cannot cope
alone.[2] Why should they be expected to face it alone? The following incident portrays the nature of the problem as seen by a
clinical instructor in medical and surgical nursing.

> In a university school of nursing careful plans were made to
> introduce students to the care of patients through a succession of
> steps beginning with the least disturbing. Since death was considered
> the most traumatic, the school hoped that students might be able to
> avoid contact with it until they had been helped in "working
> through" their feelings about a considerable number of less difficult
> situations. Because death does not accept the imposition of time
> schedules, some five girls about eighteen years old were suddenly
> faced with its reality long before they had had all the preparation
> the school hoped to give them.
>
> They threw themselves down on the floor in an available room,
> and in the presence of their clinical instructor "they wept, and wept,
> and wept." Their sobbing was very upsetting to her because she did
> not know what to do to comfort them. The only thing she could

[1] Wertenbaker, Lael Tucker, *Death of a Man*. Random House, New York, 1957,
p. 57.

[2] In "A Case-Study in the Functioning of Social Systems as a Defence Against
Anxiety: A Report of the Nursing Service of a General Hospital," appearing in
Human Relations, vol. 13, no. 2, 1960, pp. 95–120, Isabel E. P. Menzies concludes that
over the long course of the British hospital's history, nursing has unconsciously
evolved an elaborate social system designed to protect nurses against anxiety. As a
result, most of them rarely have more than brief and superficial contacts with any
one patient. A portion of this case study has been reproduced as Appendix 6.

think of was that they must be permitted to cry; when she had been a student no visible weeping was tolerated. Afterward she decided that she must have help in learning how to give comfort. A psychiatrist, commenting on her report of a sense of inadequacy, said that she had unquestionably done the most important thing in letting the students weep and for as long as they needed. What *she* needed was help in facing her own anxiety about the students, not in learning how to comfort them.

Death is certainly not the only cause of anxiety encountered in the hospital. There may be almost as many causes as there are staff who work directly with patients. One can scarcely imagine a person who is completely free of "sore spots," but the factor that exacerbates those spots varies markedly from person to person.[1] Many of the physical conditions produced by certain diseases, or environmental situations resulting from surgery and radical treatments, may be very hard for some staff members to tolerate. Perhaps even more of the causes of anxiety do not stem from visible unpleasantness. "I don't want patients to tell me their troubles; I can't do anything to help them, and I only get upset myself" is the kind of statement that one hears repeatedly expressed or implied.

Elderly and long-term patients create frustration and annoyance for large numbers of staff. The American culture, which has tended to slough off its elderly instead of cherishing them and according them great respect as in some countries, is probably reflected in the psychosocial, if not physical, neglect of such persons that characterizes many hospitals. But this very neglect may well produce a sense of guilt.

One can hardly escape the conclusion that the hospital presents its staff with so many of those aspects of life that manifest themselves in suffering, physical and mental deterioration, and death that to neglect the worker must almost inevitably result in the neglect of the patient. We would, therefore, emphatically make greater psychological security one of the necessities of staff. As yet there is far too little knowledge of ways whereby more security can be provided under any conditions, and certainly under

[1] As illustration, see the case material interpreted by Dr. Frederick Wyatt in "Guidance Problems Among Student Nurses," *American Journal of Orthopsychiatry*, vol. 17, July, 1947, pp. 416–425.

conditions that are practical when time, numbers of staff, and costs are considered. Throughout the remainder of the monograph, however, we shall include various suggestions that appear promising, some of which have been tried with supposedly good results. In this connection the reader is referred to "The Case of the Cup Cake Treatment," reproduced as Appendix 1, which well illustrates how neglect of an elderly man was replaced by warm and interested attention first in him and then in the other patients in the geriatric unit.

THE DESIRE FOR SELF-ACTUALIZATION

Much of the foregoing discussion of psychosocial needs of staff might have been presented under the broader title, the desire for self-actualization. If Dr. Argyris' thoughtful analysis has validity, this is the essence of what the individual wants from his work as well as from life generally.[1] To provide opportunity for the greatest amount of self-actualization possible becomes, therefore, the task of the hospital, as well as any other organization that hopes to minimize frustration and to maximize motivation.

No one should believe, for a moment, that an institution can make provision for it readily or easily. Even to meet the several psychosocial needs that have already been discussed must appear very burdensome to the average hospital. These needs, however, have been described in management as well as social science literature so frequently that they can scarcely be unknown to administrators. In varying degrees hospitals have attempted to meet some of them, at least for part of their staff, although not necessarily on a conceptualized or systematic basis.

But there are other psychosocial needs which may be viewed as essential components of the process of self-actualization that have not been mentioned in this chapter and that have received little attention in the literature written for administrators. From the behavioral sciences, particularly the psychology of growth and development, Dr. Argyris has assembled seven tendencies that he assumes characterize human beings in American culture. Al-

---

[1] The theme of *Personality and Organization* is the conflict between the worker's desire for self-actualization and the social system of the organization.

though some of them relate to topics already discussed, they go well beyond anything said earlier, both in breadth and in depth. More importantly they set psychosocial needs within a dynamic frame of reference in which the *developmental* aspects of personality receive merited attention as the determinants of need. The seven postulates are substantially as follows:

1. Human beings tend to develop from a state of psychological passivity as infants to a state of increasing activity as adults. This is part of the process toward development of self-initiative or self-determination.

2. Tend to develop from a state of dependence upon others as infants to a state of relative independence as adults. Relative independence is the ability to "stand on one's own two feet" and simultaneously acknowledge healthy dependencies. It is characterized by the liberation of the individual from the family that is the childhood determiner of behavior, and by the growth of one's own set of behavioral determiners. A person who has passed through this process of development successfully does not tend to react to those in positions of authority on the basis of patterns learned during childhood.

3. Tend to develop from being capable of behaving only in a few ways as an infant to being capable of behaving in many different ways as an adult.

4. Tend to develop from having interests as an infant that are erratic, shallow, and quickly dropped to having deeper interests as an adult. Maturity is characterized by endless challenges where the reward comes from doing something for its own sake, and where phenomena are analyzed and studied in their wholeness, complexity, and depth.

5. Tend to develop from a short-time perspective as an infant where the present largely determines behavior, to a much longer time perspective where behavior is more affected by the past and future. This tendency plays an important role in how workers seek to secure their future, not only economically but status-wise.

6. Tend to develop from being in a subordinate position in the family and society as an infant to aspiring to occupy an equal or superordinate position relative to their peers.

7. Tend to develop from a lack of awareness of self as an infant to an awareness of and control over self as an adult. The adult who learns to experience adequate and successful control over his own behavior is likely to develop a sense of personal integrity and feelings of self-worth.[1]

[1] Argyris, Chris, *Personality and Organization*, p. 50.

Taken together, these tendencies provide a composite description of the growth of the individual in our culture. The rate of growth and the distance traveled along each of these dimensional lines vary markedly from person to person. Some individuals progress rapidly and far; others travel slowly and cover relatively short distances. Were a clinical psychologist or a psychiatrist to attempt to make a profile of where an individual stands at a given time, the graph would probably indicate great unevenness of development. Self-actualization may be thought of as the individual's plotted score along the above dimensions.

For an understanding of the probable satisfactions and dissatisfactions of persons who work in complex organizations such as hospitals, a knowledge of these tendencies is essential. The normal growth pattern suggests that to the degree to which workers achieve emotional maturity, they will need the chance to express independence and autonomy, make decisions that determine the outcome of their efforts, participate in significant relationships with their equals, and perhaps advance to supervisory or executive positions. If the institution can provide such opportunities, the "fit" between it and them should be good. If, on the other hand, work situations foster passiveness, dependency, and subordination of role, the "fit" may produce acute discomfort.

The next chapter on small work groups, interpolated because the subject warrants more attention than could be given it earlier, will underscore the significance of this particular kind of opportunity for self-actualization. Subsequent chapters will permit some evaluation of the extent to which self-actualization is fostered or hindered by the formal organization of the hospital and its resulting social system.

Chapter 2

SMALL WORK GROUPS

EARLIER REFERENCE was made to the potential importance of the worker's immediate peer group in his quest for social approval and a sense of significance in what he is doing. The peer group offers him not only this support but so much more that it becomes essential to include informal membership in such a group as a psychosocial requirement for most employees.[1]

Small work groups, furthermore, are of major importance to the organizational design and the on-going program of an institution, and must be examined from that perspective, too. Consequently, this chapter is devoted exclusively to the subject of small work groups, or primary groups as they would also be designated by social scientists. They will be viewed first in their role of contributing to staff security, support, and opportunity for social contacts. They will be viewed secondly as constituting the informal organization of the institution, capable of setting work norms and exercising considerable indirect power over administration.[2] We shall then be ready in the next chapter to begin examination of the formal organization.

WORK GROUPS IN THEIR BENEFIT TO EMPLOYEES

Any large institution is so truly vast, complex, and stratified that personnel in relatively central positions have difficulty in

[1] It must be clearly understood that the group referred to here is of the kind where interpersonal relations already exist among its members. Much experimental study has been devoted to "small groups," composed generally of graduate students or other individuals employed for this purpose, who had not previously established acquaintanceship and communication and hence were not groups at all as the term is employed in this context.

[2] "The Informal Organization of Industry" in Dr. J. A. C. Brown's *The Social Psychology of Industry* (Penguin Books, Inc., Baltimore, 1958, pp. 124–157) is a fine synthesis of what had been learned up to 1954 about small work groups in both of these aspects. Many of the ideas presented here have been taken from this chapter.

knowing enough about its purposes, goals, and current programs to feel a close identification with it. For administrators to assume that those in less favored positions can or will try to gain a sense of belonging to it psychologically—even though they be given talks and literature—has not been borne out by many of the studies made. Most persons tend to identify themselves with a relatively small number of other persons and frequently with those who are close at hand. Thus employees may become informal members of several small and often overlapping groups within the institution that serve a variety of purposes. Such groups appear, moreover, on every level from assistant directors to "kitchen help."

Where mobility is limited by the nature of the job, spatial proximity becomes so important that the worker's strongest social contacts generally coincide with his immediate work group. This fact has great significance for ward or floor staffs. Persons like nursing supervisors or medical residents, who are spatially separated by their work, may be able to maintain regularly constituted small groups at coffee breaks or during meals in the cafeteria. Formal observations have revealed the consistency with which the same persons sit together in hospital dining rooms, and the hesitation of anyone else to take a needed chair that happens to be vacant.

Small work groups, like other primary groups, rarely average more than eight or ten persons. Beyond that size face-to-face communication becomes difficult, and the group is likely to split into two units. These units provide their members with an opportunity for more than mere acquaintanceship: for laughing and joking, "blowing off steam" about "the boss" or the evils of the world in general, keeping each other in hand, congratulating or sympathizing with one another. Here Eddie tells Jack that he is about to be married or that his father is not going to live; here Mary confides to her friends that her daughter is pregnant and she will become a grandmother.

Members of the group may like, dislike, or be indifferent to other members, but relationships are direct and each person generally knows how he feels toward the others. If given a sociometric test, members can usually indicate the persons who most clearly express the attitudes and beliefs of the group and who are, therefore, what the sociologists call the *norm bearers*. Relationships within the group are in sharp contrast to the formality and cautiousness exhibited toward representatives of administration who constitute what is often called the secondary group.

The status accorded each member of the in-group is not primarily determined by the work he does, but rests upon the considerable knowledge that the group has of him. One man may have a highly developed skill useful to his job that is greatly admired; another may have skill in playing cards or fishing that is equally admired. A third worker proves to be the member of the group who keeps everyone laughing, or simply "a good Joe" who is spontaneously liked, or the person who listens sympathetically to others' troubles. Perhaps he is the one best able "to run interference" for the group with the boss. There are so many ways in which to achieve status within the small group that almost everyone can have the sense of belongingness without the external signs of status which organizations use in the hope of giving their employees that sense.

If groups are stable enough to become well integrated, their activities may extend beyond the place of work or take on an appearance of exclusiveness. Some of the members perhaps develop the habit of bowling or going to ball games together. An occasional picnic or a dinner in a downtown restaurant celebrates a birthday or coming wedding. Little group mannerisms and idiosyncratic words and phrases begin to appear, whereby members indicate to themselves and to others that they belong to an in-group which in some way is different from and superior to every other group. Not infrequently a new person assigned to the work unit is given "a rough time" before he is received into the in-group.

Perhaps because the small work group repeats so many of the characteristics of that prototype of all primary groups, the family, it appears to meet a need felt by all except a few "isolates." Like the family it is founded on a desire for security, social satisfactions, and personal relationships; and it seeks to maintain itself as a unity.

As illustration of how important a role small groups may play in providing psychological support in times of adversity, we present a résumé of a story told the writer by a faculty member of a university school of nursing. This instructor had had her basic training in a hospital school that, in midcentury, still reproduced the military aspects of nursing education of an earlier period. The rigidity and even punitiveness of the director's office appeared also to characterize many members of the teaching staff.

A class of sixty students had scarcely been admitted to the school when they were told repetitively, "The door swings out as well as in." What that statement meant was made abundantly clear on the evening of the "capping ceremony" when the sixty girls stood up to receive their nursing caps in the presence of representatives of the hospital and invited relatives and friends. One half of them received no caps. Without specific warning they were dropped from the school in a public ceremony, on an occasion generally regarded as the happiest in the nursing students' career. The other half received their caps while choking down sobs when they saw what was happening.

During their subsequent clinical experience, the remaining thirty students had to meet one anxiety-inducing situation after another without any sympathy or understanding interest being shown them. Every student was expected to face the trauma of incurable disease and death without visible sign of emotion. When the writer inquired how it had been possible for these girls in late adolescence to come through such an experience without serious scars or extended psychiatric treatment, the instructor said that she attributed survival to the efficacy of small groups. She described the group of some eight students to which she had belonged who clung together in sheer desperation. They were so supporting of one another in the face of common danger that she decided later that they had been their own and each other's therapists.

PROBLEMS OF MAINTAINING SMALL GROUPS IN HOSPITALS

From the foregoing it would seem almost imperative that the hospital foster the development of small groups because of the help they can often give their members. Unfortunately, many groups, regardless of their location, are not stable enough to have any prolonged existence. Well-integrated groups appear most frequently in firmly established industries, businesses, and institutions employing skilled workers or technically and professionally trained personnel, and in relatively small and long established communities. Where labor turnover is high, workers are employed on a part-time basis, or employees are rotated or moved from one unit to another, small groups have great difficulty in

maintaining themselves intact. These very factors of high turnover, part-time work, and rotation, which are deterrents to the
development of successful small groups, characterize so many
hospitals that they must receive further attention.

Hospitals having resident house staffs generally deem themselves fortunate when compared with those numerous institutions
that must depend almost exclusively upon physicians in private
practice for their medical service. The pattern of the full-time,
closed or partially closed staff of senior physicians, characteristic
of European general hospitals, has rarely existed in the United
States. Generally it is found only in hospitals serving special
groups in the population such as those under the management of
the federal government or the United Mine Workers' Union. In
hospitals accredited for internships and residencies, the house
staff of junior physicians come for a designated period, generally
of one to three years. This fact, combined with the requirement
of frequent rotation, seriously weakens the opportunity for the
development of well-integrated small groups. Such groups might
be exceedingly useful to their members at the very time when
young doctors are faced with uncertainty and anxiety not only
about medical diagnosis and treatment, but about their role and
place within the authority structure of the institution. Their uncertainties are often reflected in their strained relations with
nurses, and in their harried impersonal relations with patients to
which reference has been made.

Similar problems are encountered in nursing. Large numbers
of undergraduate nursing students and increasing numbers of
nurses enrolled for graduate study spend limited periods participating in nursing care on the various clinical services of hospitals.
These students can scarely become integral parts of work groups.
They may themselves not seriously need the help of such groups
since they are probably members of well-established groups in
their school, and are frequently assisted generously in the hospital
by a clinical instructor. But their frequent coming and going
deters the development of stable group relations among the
regular staff.

Let us look now at turnover as that term is conventionally used.
Because of shortages of nursing personnel, large hospitals progres-

sively use various methods of recruitment that seem to promise increased numbers of applicants although it is recognized that turnover is likely to be high. Educational and cultural advantages, opportunity to enjoy a big city or sea or mountains, to travel to distant parts of the United States, or to gain experience in highly specialized and new clinical fields are featured as inducements from which hospitals of great distinction or in desired spots profit at least briefly. Recruitment, however, has become so competitive and the inducements often so glowing that, once the newness of a position and place has worn off, many nurses decide to move on to supposedly greener pastures. Hence these very efforts have been serious handicaps to the making of stable teams for patient care that could provide some guarantee of continuity and efficiency of service.

A director of nursing service recently pointed to a thirty per cent annual turnover among her large staff of graduate nurses. For the small number of practical nurses employed the figure was five per cent; for the aides who were largest in number and predominantly men, the figure was one per cent. She cited all the advantages of the particular city as reasons for nurses or their husbands being attracted to it. But, said she, when the husbands have finished their graduate work or their medical residencies, the nurses will leave to go wherever the family decides to settle. And, of course, some of them will have children in the meantime and will have to leave at least temporarily. How is it possible, she and other directors query, to have highly functioning nursing teams when the central figure in the work group is often in the process of arriving or of leaving, or her position is vacant?

Again because of the shortage of nurses the practice of part-time employment has become common. Nurses are engaged to supplement the regular staff at hours when work is heaviest or floor coverage the poorest. Those willing to work on weekends are especially in demand. Some nurses who have had to be away from their profession because of small children or sick family members, are delighted to be able to return even on a part-time basis. They identify themselves as quickly and completely as possible with the nursing unit. For probably a much larger number the part-time work is not their major interest, or the hours when they are present are the very ones when the work group is smallest and weakest. As a consequence they are unlikely to become fully participating members of any social group.

Rotation of regular nursing staff presents a particularly serious deterrent to the maintenance of group bonds. On many nursing units the number of persons giving direct patient care on the morning and often on the evening shift is almost ideal for constituting a small group. In spite of social differences between the graduate nurses, practical nurses, and aides, small groups might often evolve that would furnish both staff and patients much satisfaction, support high morale, and contribute to work effectiveness.

But hospitals have to be staffed the entire twenty-four hours every day in the year. Since the evening work hours (from about three to eleven o'clock) are very unpopular and night hours and weekends scarcely less so, rotation of all nurses on a systematic basis was long considered the solution most fair to staff that would guarantee coverage. The method is still used with little modification in some places. However, many hospitals now attempt to give personnel, perhaps after a preliminary period or as openings become available, their first choice of service and shift. If an adequate staffing pattern cannot be achieved in this way with the supplementary help of part-time nurses, it becomes necessary to assign personnel to vital posts. Assignment is generally made with the understanding that the worker will have to stay only a limited time on an unwanted shift or service.

Some hospitals employ a few "floating nurses" who are not attached to a particular unit but are available on call where needed. Sometimes they spend an entire shift on one unit; again they may help with several emergencies in different parts of the institution. "Floaters" are such a valuable source of relief when difficulties arise that administrators of nursing service are frequently asked why they do not employ more. The answer is simple. Most nurses thoroughly dislike "floating" and hence will not take such a position. They even dislike being sent to a unit other than their own except infrequently and for something very unusual.

Obviously the requirements of creating and maintaining an adequate staffing pattern present an almost insoluble problem for many hospitals. It is little wonder that directors of nursing service often fail to think of other aspects of the problem than how to get the requisite number of persons for the three shifts, and simultaneously make provision for a five-day work week, vacations, and sick leave. The break in an unmodified system of rotation, which almost precluded small group development, has probably come quite as much through nurses' refusal to work at hours and on services other than those designated by themselves as through any comprehensive examination of the psychosocial needs of staff.

The subject of lack of small group development, however, is one of vital significance. In it may be found some of the causes not only for high turnover, but for general dissatisfaction and an unwillingness to make much emotional commitment to the broader aspects of patient care. The following illustration suggests a probable correlation between a well-integrated nursing group and highly motivated attention to patients. General hospitals that are in a position to engage in experimental studies might well put this subject high on their research agenda.

> An experienced psychiatric nurse reported to the writer that she offered her services as a head nurse, for one year on the evening shift, to a large and excellent psychiatric hospital, provided it would not rotate any of the nursing staff on the ward and would not transfer patients to or from other units. She was willing to accept this particular shift in order to have her mornings free for graduate work in a neighboring university. Although the hospital had a policy of modified rotation of staff and transfer of patients as they improved or regressed, it was so pleased to be able to obtain her services that it decided to let her experiment with a stable situation. According to her evaluation at the end of the year, the experience had been a profitable one for everybody. Staff had learned to work together comfortably and well and constituted a true work group; staff and patients had become acquainted with each other as never before; evening programs in which both staff and patients participated had been developed; and many of these long-term schizophrenic men appeared to have moved toward higher levels of social responsibility.

THE INFORMAL ORGANIZATION OF THE INSTITUTION

The earlier sections of this chapter have dealt with the psychological profits small groups are able to confer on their members, and the difficulty hospitals encounter in permitting such groups to develop. Now the emphasis shifts to small groups as the informal organization of the institution.[1] Every institution may be thought of as composed of many such groups, existing on all levels of the hierarchical structure, and held together in some state of equilibrium by management, or administration, to use the terminology of the hospital. What roles small groups play *vis-à-vis* administration and how they are able to play these roles become, therefore, crucial questions for examination.

Since the nature and success of the roles are dependent upon the degree of integration achieved by the group, some further remarks are needed about cohesion. It has already been noted that, if groups survive, they evolve. The bonds that unite or sustain their members tend to increase in strength until the group becomes an entity that is something more than a collection of individuals.[2] Simultaneously stable characteristics develop that are hard to change. Not until certain characteristics have appeared, however, is the group strong enough to become an effective social unit. Structure must be sufficiently well defined for each person to have a place in the group and to know what to expect from everyone else; interaction among the members is a necessity; and leadership within the group must have emerged to a degree that permits the making and carrying out of plans.

In a recent study Captain Robert H. Cortner sought to prove the hypothesis that the morale of any small task-oriented group is relative to the knowledge the group has of its own informal group structure.[3] From his examination of the attitudes of thirty work groups on all levels in two hospitals, he found that high-morale groups selected "group leaders" significantly more often than low-morale groups; they chose one from the group as "best on the job" significantly more often; and they selected an individual as representing the group's "contact with hospital administration," whereas low-morale groups did not.

[1] Preiss, Jack J., "The Phenomena of Informal Organization," *Hospital Administration*, vol. 4, Spring, 1959, pp. 35–45.

[2] Strauss, George, and Leonard R. Sayles, *Personnel: The Human Problems of Management*, Prentice-Hall, Inc., Englewood Cliffs, N. J., 1960, p. 62. Readers are referred to Chapter 3, Work Groups and Informal Organization, from which many of the generalizations used in this section have been drawn.

[3] "Morale and Group Structure: The Relation Between Morale and Informal Group Structure in Hospitals." A Ph.D. dissertation submitted to St. Louis University, 1961, p. 2.

As part of the process of developing the characteristics essential for exercising power over the institution, groups must necessarily discipline their own members. Thus they serve as an important instrument for social control over employees of all categories. Members are expected not to get far out of line with group behavior. If they do, ridicule or other forms of pressure will be exerted to enforce conformity. In some instances the leeway for deviance from group norms is so slight that it would be unwise for a supervisor to try to reward an individual rather than the group. The individual might well find himself rejected. For a member to break the unwritten law of the in-group about "squealing" on a fellow employee to some one in the out-group, particularly a supervisor, merits the sharpest scorn. Even an exhibition of too much enthusiasm for one's job may be frowned upon, unless the group has indicated that increased interest is permissible, lest it "show up" the other employees. The simple incident reported here illustrates how little escapes group scrutiny.

> A nursing aide came into a patient's room one evening almost dancing, and with eyes sparkling. When the patient commented that she seemed to be "well up," the aide replied, "Some of the girls [the other aides on the floor] tell me I shouldn't say so, but I love to work in a hospital. I love to make patients feel as comfortable as I can." This aide was recognized by the patients as a remarkable person whose very presence made them feel better. Anyone walking along the corridor could frequently hear them calling for her by name. When her remark was repeated to a social scientist acquainted with the hospital, the latter said instantly, "She should not let the other aides hear her say that she loves to work in a hospital. If she does, she is likely to get into trouble."

The group expects its members to do their fair share of the work, and also help each other when the need arises; no person, however, should do too much. Often the group determines what is a "fair day's work" and keeps production within the range of the average worker.[1] Thus it sets the work norm referred to earlier. As Max Weber, the German sociologist pointed out many years ago, "restriction of production" has long been a natural

[1] See the telling illustration reproduced as Appendix 2.

and almost universal phenomenon. Great ability has been shown in resisting the demands of industrial management for additional output, longer work hours, and higher quality. Under some conditions, however, such as competitiveness between groups, eagerness to demonstrate what can be achieved or willingness to help meet emergency situations, the group decides that levels of effort should be high. Pace can be drastically altered by a determined group. It may be assumed that the situation is similar in hospitals: if adequate observations could be made by the administration, it might sometimes be discovered on the lower hierarchical levels that the staff were not too few in number but that they were skillfully controlling how much work should be done.

Usually power is directed by the group against the immediate supervisor. Therefore, supervisors often realize that although they have the authority to make many decisions, it is frequently unwise to exercise that authority. "The members of the group can express their displeasure by cutting down their work pace, sabotaging the work (discreetly, of course, so that blame will be hard to place), or making their boss look inept to his own supervisors. This is probably the most potent form of protection that the group can offer its members."[1]

> Food trays were brought to patients in a particular hospital by men from the food service who collected them as soon as the meal was finished. If the dishes needed to be sterilized, however, that task was the responsibility of the nursing aides. A patient, whose dishes were to be washed separately, could not understand why her tray was generally left in her room from one to three hours, even after she had requested over the "intercom" system to have it removed. She concluded that the aides disliked to sterilize dishes in spite of the excellent equipment available, because they did not consider it a part of their regular duties. When she mentioned the problem one day to the head nurse who had inquired whether there was anything she would like, the nurse's reply was strangely vague; the dishes continued to remain in her room. Later the social scientist referred to earlier explained that "the nurses" were careful to keep the aides "pacified." Hence even the head nurse with complete authority had undoubtedly refrained from requesting action.

[1] Strauss, George, and Leonard R. Sayles, *Personnel: The Human Problems of Management*, p. 60.

HOSPITAL ADMINISTRATION AND SMALL WORK GROUPS

Obviously cohesive, well-disciplined small groups have the ability to wield a surprising amount of power.[1] They can use this power either to contribute to or impede the effectiveness of the institution. They contribute only "when the standards of behavior they enforce are articulated with the requirements of formal authority."[2] As a consequence it is of paramount importance that administration should try to find ways and means to make its aims and goals and those of the work groups conform to the highest degree possible.

Industry and business long disliked and feared small groups, and frequently tried to destroy them or retard their development. Employees responded by being recalcitrant, exigent in their demands, and by resorting to force if necessary, particularly if they were members of trade unions that determined when and how physical power should be applied. Under such conditions management often confused small group behavior with that of mobs or crowds, whose potential reactions are always terrifying for the very reason that a system of interpersonal relations and group control is lacking.

In recent years industrial and business management has become progressively aware that it must know far more about the group behavior of workers, and must make perhaps drastic alterations in its relations with employees. Otherwise it cannot even hope to win their support in the setting and achieving of common work goals. Graduate schools of industrial relations or business administration have busied themselves with publishing materials that would give management a better understanding of its role; personnel psychologists and sometimes psychiatrists have been attached to many plants; short training courses in "human relations" have become very popular, and have been attended particularly by representatives of middle management from the supposedly progressive firms.

[1] See Robert N. Wilson's splendid article, "The Primary Group in the Hospital" (*Hospital Administration*, vol. 3, Summer, 1958, pp. 13–23), in which he views closely coordinated, small work groups as probably "the most important locus of decision in the hospital."

[2] Janowitz, Morris, *Sociology and the Military Establishment*. Russell Sage Foundation, New York, 1959, p. 65.

Interestingly the military establishment, which had been viewed as conservative and inflexible, began to sponsor extensive social science research during World War II relating to motives and attitudes as aspects of military life.[1] The results pointed clearly to the crucial role played in combat effectiveness by strong small group loyalty. "Thinking that you couldn't let the other men in your outfit down" was second only to prayer, according to selected combat troops who were asked to comment on what thoughts were helpful "when the going was rough."[2] An infantry scout who had fought through Sicily summarized the intense loyalty to one's "buddies" and its meaning for the individual in the words, "You know the men in your outfit. You have to be loyal to them. The men get close-knit together. They like each other—quit their petty bickering and having enemies. They depend on each other—wouldn't do anything to let the rest of them down. They'd rather be killed than do that. They begin to think a world of each other. It's the main thing that keeps a man from going haywire."[3] Studies showed that even in totalitarian armies primary group solidarity was an unmistakable source of military efficiency.

When the results of this research became available for examination, their potential importance made a strong impression on some segments of industry and business. Many corporations are now continuing attitude studies of a similar kind as a tool of administrative management.

Hospital administration is also beginning to follow the trend of increased interest in discovering what makes people within the institutional setting willing or unwilling to work, and how human resources can be utilized for greater effectiveness. Progressively larger attention is being given to these questions through teaching and research in departments of hospital administration, which are generally parts of schools of public health, and through articles appearing particularly in *Hospital Administration*, published by the American College of Hospital Administrators. The American College, moreover, sponsors an annual award for the book chosen

---

[1] Stouffer, Samuel A., and others, *The American Soldier*. Princeton University Press, Princeton, N. J., 1949. 4 vols.

[2] *Ibid.*, vol. 2, p. 177.

[3] *Ibid.*, vol. 2, p. 137.

by one of its committees that appears to make a significant contribution to administration in general.

No one should assume, however, that the average general hospital has any considerable knowledge of the psychosocial aspects of work groups; their potential significance in determining the quantity and quality of patient care; or how the goals of administration (including physicians as supervisors of patient care) and those of the ward staff who provide direct care can be harmonized. Hospitals appear to be highly conservative institutions where attention is still far more focused on the hierarchical than upon the informal structure.

In comparison with industry and business fewer representatives of hospital administration or of medical staffs, except for some individual psychiatrists, seem to have informed themselves about social science literature and experiments dealing with pertinent subjects such as group attitudes, communication, motivation, and group counseling. Nurses in surprising numbers have attended short training courses in human relations, but as yet these courses have perhaps served more to strengthen the ego of the nurse than to produce change in the clinical setting. Instances, like those cited earlier of ward staffs seeking to get through the work day as easily as possible even at the expense of patient comfort, are indicative of administration's failure to reach such groups with a dynamic program designed to meet their psychological needs and simultaneously those of patients.

In its Summer, 1961, issue, the *Journal of Health and Human Behavior* included the article, "Control Over Policy by Attendants in a Mental Hospital," written by Dr. Thomas J. Scheff, a sociologist who had spent six months observing four wards of a state institution. For the administrative and medical staff of long-term institutions where the attendant personnel are relatively stable and well entrenched, this article would appear to be almost indispensable reading. It is cited here because its theoretical frame of reference, and particularly its description of the techniques used by the attendants for gaining control over policy, might be illuminating to many administrators of general hospitals. Although no recapitulation can be given in this brief monograph of the techniques employed, Dr. Scheff's "Summary" on pages 104–105 is quoted to indicate the assumptions drawn from his observations.

"This analysis of the reaction of the staff of a large mental hospital to an administrative program of change has revolved around the question, how was the staff able to resist the program introduced by the administration? It suggests that the answer lay in the differing structures of the administrative and staff groups.

"The staff of the hospital was a stable and highly organized community. Within this community, over the years, an informal system of sanctions and rationalizations had evolved. They enabled the staff to exert control over the administration and to keep discipline within its own ranks. The system of social control was sufficiently effective to stalemate a vigorous program of reform introduced by the administration. The system was also so pervasive that even the sizable group within the staff who wished to participate in hospital reform were confused or neutralized.

"The administrative and medical personnel, by contrast, were highly mobile and lacking in the training and interest necessary to provide leadership in the staff community. Because of the shortages of personnel and resources, and the nature of the physicians' training, the administration relied largely on formal controls, without the informal system of controls which usually supports changes in organizations. In this situation, the defensive tactics of the staff were effective to the point that the program did not reach completion."

METHODS OF WORKING WITH STAFF GROUPS

Subsequent chapters will suggest further reasons why programs designed to harmonize the goals of the administration and those of the informal groups have been so late in appearing in general hospitals. (Regardless of the discouraging nature of Dr. Scheff's report, a considerable number of psychiatric institutions have made distinctive advances.) Some of the later discussion concerning improvement of patient care through more effective relationships among staff, moreover, will be directly applicable to small groups. Without waiting until those parts of the text have been reached, we now wish to describe one program and the contents of one talk that deal specifically, and on a relatively high level of sophistication, with how administrative and supervisory personnel, including physicians, can work with groups of ward staff to achieve common goals. We regret being obliged to draw upon undertakings from psychiatric rather than general hospitals, but we believe that the applicability of many of the assumptions and methods will be apparent.

"An Aide-Centered Activity Program for Elderly Patients," as it was called, was initiated at Winter Veterans Administration Hospital in Topeka, Kansas, an institution primarily for neuropsychiatric patients but with a large general medical and surgical service.[1] A reevaluation of care on the unit for elderly patients indicated that physical needs were being well met, but emotional needs of individual patients required concentrated attention. Since nursing aides, or nursing assistants as the V.A. calls them for purposes of increased recognition, are with the patients far more than anyone else, the question was one of how they could be motivated and helped to assume responsibility that extended well beyond the daily physical care of their charges.

The nursing supervisor suggested to the assistants that they might like to learn more about the total patient-care program for this group of senile, if not psychotic, men. Hence they were given time to visit the physical and corrective therapy units where they could find out about the objectives of treatment of those two services. The nursing supervisor met with them regularly to provide opportunity for discussion of what they had learned, as well as discussion of their own skills and interests.

At about this time a questionnaire was designed to survey quickly the different skills and interests of each nurse and nursing assistant. Under Sports, Hobbies or Special Interest, Table Games, and Reading, a large number of specific items were listed. Each of these items was to be checked in one of the three columns labeled Active, Would Like to Learn, No Interest. The completed questionnaires were viewed as a prospective aid not only in assigning the most interested personnel to the various activities on and off the unit, but in stimulating initiative among the ward staff in wanting to organize patient groups.

The focus of the meetings led by the nursing supervisor then became one of encouraging the assistants to plan, develop, and expand patient activities in their own way but in close relationship with their charges. The objective of these activities was described to the assistants as "helping the patient to share group experiences." Attention was also focused upon encouraging the assistants to see and think about the patients as individuals.

---

[1] This description has been prepared from the unpublished paper, "An Aide Centered Activity Program for Elderly Patients," and from a brief visit made by the writer to the program. The authors of the paper are James Folsom, Jacob Gier, and Llewellyn White, two of the physicians and the nursing supervisor referred to in the text.

At the request of the nursing supervisor her meetings with the assistants were replaced by those of a Rehabilitation Team, whose purpose was to demonstrate the importance of the assistant as a member of the treatment group and to overcome his reluctance to talk and to share in the planning of activities. All the members of a complete rehabilitation team, as constituted in the Winter V.A. Hospital, attended the meetings whenever they could. They included the chief psychiatrist of the Geriatrics Section, the internist for the Section, the chief of the Physical Medicine and Rehabilitation Service who is a psychiatrist, the nurses and nursing assistants of the unit, a social worker, occupational therapist, corrective therapist, physical therapist, librarian, recreational leader, and volunteer worker.

The nursing assistants were asked to suggest activities they would like to start with patients, such as ceramics, yard work, or singing. They then received initial assistance in planning from the appropriate adjunctive therapists, and began working with small groups of patients under the supervision of these therapists. If they exhibited sufficient interest and ability, they were shortly encouraged to use their own initiative in creating activity programs. As a result patients, who had spent much of their time sitting idly in the dayroom or pacing the floor aggressively because of inadequate numbers of occupational and recreational therapists, were introduced to a variety of group undertakings on the unit, out-of-doors, or in the hospital shops.

The meetings of the Rehabilitation Team were also used to emphasize the potential value of every staff-patient relationship. Furthermore, they provided a place where assistants were invited to bring their problems with individual patients. Among these senile men irritability, agitation, hyperactivity, noisiness, or even assaultiveness were not uncommon and created difficult management situations. Through group discussion ways could often be found for reducing a patient's tension, thus making things more comfortable for him, the other men, and the assistants. The very opportunity to express frustration and anxiety in a sympathetic group tended, moreover, to reduce stress among the assistants.

In the opinion of the physicians and the nursing supervisor, the principal value of this program lay in its recognition of the importance of the nursing assistant as a member of a total treatment group; in its according him status through the meetings of the Rehabilitation Team; and in his then assuming his place in the overall planning of patient activities.

Interesting considerations are raised by this ambitious undertaking. One may assume that the nursing supervisor had already accomplished much in helping the assistants develop within an accepted small group, and that they already knew and felt relatively comfortable with the physicians who visited the unit, as they did with her. They had been given time and opportunity to explore the treatment offered by physical and corrective therapy, and to indicate their own skills and interests; these opportunities they may have perceived as forms of recognition.

Had there been no such developmental process, would they have viewed the meetings of the Rehabilitation Team as an acknowledgment of their potential importance to the institution? Or would they have viewed these sessions as another administrative scheme for getting them to do more work? Even if they had wanted to be active participants in the Team meetings, would they have felt comfortable enough to talk in a fairly large group composed primarily of status figures and professionally trained persons?

In an unpublished talk given in the late 1950s, Dr. John Cumming drew upon his knowledge of sociology and social psychology, and his valuable experience as an administrative psychiatrist in working closely with ward staffs and nursing supervisors in two hospitals.[1] Thus he attempted to find possible answers to just such questions in order that administrators may avoid some of the pitfalls frequently encountered when they attempt to encourage small work groups to raise levels of patient care.

Many physicians have appreciable difficulty in working closely with nursing personnel. According to Dr. Cumming's thesis, however, those who carry administrative responsibility for patient care have no alternative if the limited staffs of the average psychiatric hospital are to be used to best advantage. Since the small ward group sets the work norms, the doctor must realize that change can be achieved only through interaction with that group. Hence he must be prepared—or prepare himself—to become an interacting member of the ward staff.

How to gain entrée into the group is a vital question. Through interesting himself in the problems faced by the nurses and aides in the ward setting and trying to assist them, doors will generally be opened to him. One of the easiest ways for the doctor to enter the ward culture is informally, perhaps by being around at the coffee break and using any casual opportunity for talking to the

---

[1] "The Rehabilitation of Chronic Patients in Mental Hospitals," pp. 4–9.

nurses, learning their problems, interests, and opinions. Later when he knows them better, this time can be extended to regularly scheduled ward meetings.

Often the physician has responsibility for so many wards in a hospital that it is not possible for him to spend the requisite time with the staff of one unit. Under these circumstances Dr. Cumming recommends that the physician work with representatives from several wards who, in turn, will work with their own groups. In this process it is essential that the nursing personnel of the several wards play a large role in determining who should represent them. Were the doctor to make the selection, he would naturally choose persons whose attitudes he liked; if the representatives are selected by the members of the small groups they will probably be the norm bearers of those groups. By the process of selection, moreover, they have been given permission "to go out and get new information." These facts greatly increase the likelihood that the small groups will accept "the information" brought back.

In conducting meetings that center around problems of patient care, Dr. Cumming suggests that the physician refrain from "delivering lectures" or talking extensively. Instead, he needs from the very beginning to address by name the persons with the lowest prestige in the group, and ask them for facts or opinions based upon their observations. Otherwise the meetings are likely to be a conversation between the doctor and the one or two senior persons who attend. It may even be desirable initially not to invite nurses on the supervisory level.

When all the details about the situation brought up for discussion have been assembled, it will often be obvious to everyone that the incident had certain understandable causes, and ways for preventing its recurrence will become clear. In the early days of these meetings the approval of the physician is one of the chief motivating forces that keeps the group searching for solutions. Subsequently, problem-solving in itself will come to be of value to the group and they will not rely so heavily on interpersonal rewards from him. Later, moreover, when staffs request additional information and guidance that will be of general use to them in problem-solving, the physician may drop his role of group leader and become a teacher.

Chapter 3

THE FORMAL STRUCTURE OF THE
GENERAL HOSPITAL

THE PRECEDING CHAPTER has attempted to demonstrate the significance of interpersonal relations as manifested through what they can accomplish in providing psychological support to the members of face-to-face groups, and in exerting pressure on the institution even when the groups are not backed by unions or vigorous professional associations. Ever since Harry Stack Sullivan developed the psychiatric theory of interpersonal relations, it has found increasing favor among psychiatrists and social scientists, not only in its application to situations between therapist and individual patient but as a method capable of producing changes in group attitudes and behavior. It has been made the basis of much of the work in group dynamics and human relations that has already exerted considerable influence both in management and in labor circles. As a consequence many persons interested in seeing the motivation and competence of personnel raised in behalf of greater productivity (in this instance, of better patient care) almost take it for granted that if interpersonal relations can be strengthened in positive ways the major problem will be solved.

This assumption appears to those who have examined the formal structure of large-scale organizations as much too optimistic. Important as are work groups, any complex undertaking, whether it be industry, business, the federal government, or the expanded hospital, is organized on bureaucratic or hierarchical lines.[1] This very type of structure works against, and often almost

[1] See Marjorie Taubenhaus' amusing article, "Hospital Hierarchy," which appears as Appendix 3.

56

precludes, the creation and maintenance of sufficient channels for acquaintanceship and informal communication, through which interpersonal relationships could develop to produce effective results. Because so much effort is being spent at present by the health services in cultivating the theory and practice of interpersonal relations and so little relatively in studying the nature and behavioral consequences of the formal structure, some careful scrutiny must be given to the hierarchical system of the general hospital.

THE HOSPITAL'S ORGANIZATION CHART

Like other operating agencies concerned with the production and distribution of goods or services, hospitals have learned to draw diagrams, known as organization charts, to indicate the formal structure of the institution. These charts are a kind of statement in shorthand of the pattern of rules according to which the regular tasks of the organization are to be carried out, and the members of the organization ideally relate to each other in task-performance.[1] Thus they are a picture that supposedly can be read by anyone accustomed to examining such charts, of the way in which it is expected that things will be done. Inherent in them are characteristics of the value system of American culture: responsibility, authority and command, status, prestige, obedience, and submission.

Although organization charts vary from hospital to hospital in many minor details, the accompanying diagram suggests the pattern of major relationships that one might expect to find in a large institution. A hypothetical teaching hospital of more than 500 beds, not owned by a university, has been selected for portrayal because it has professional personnel on all levels of responsibility and authority, in addition to a great diversity of technically trained and untrained staff. Had a hospital of 150 beds been chosen, the organization chart would have shown fewer departments or services and the "chain of command" would have been shorter. For the very reason that many hospitals still continue to

[1] Henry, Jules, "The Formal Social Structure of a Psychiatric Hospital," *Psychiatry*, vol. 17, May, 1954, p. 140. This excellent article by Dr. Henry has been utilized extensively in the preparation of these pages.

ORGANIZATION CHART OF A LARGE TEACHING HOSPITAL[a]

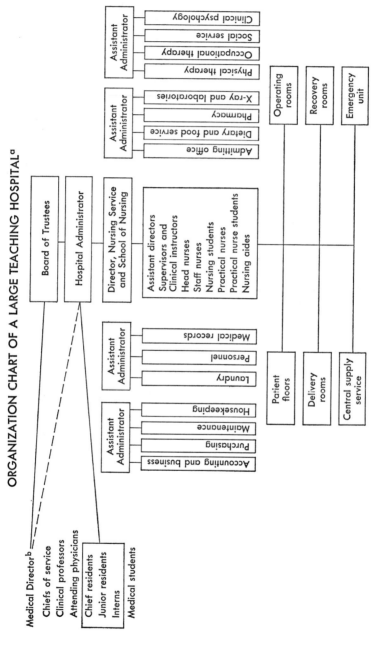

[a] No attempt has been made on this rough chart to separate service and educational functions, or to show their exact organizational relationships to each other and to hospital administration. Nor has the school of nursing administration been included in the diagram.

[b] Several different terms may be used to designate the person who is the clinical head of a medical service; the most common is chief of staff. In this instance the full-time salaried head is designated as the medical director; he carries administrative and clinical responsibility for medical care of patients and medical education and research. Had this hospital been owned by a university, the dean of the medical school probably would have been the head of the medical service, and he might also have been the administrative head of the hospital; the chiefs of service customarily would have been the chairmen of the school's clinical departments.

become progressively larger, while size multiplies administrative problems, our discussion will be confined to large institutions.

At the top of the chart is the designation of the overall governing body, generally known as a board of trustees or directors. If the hospital is a voluntary one, as in this instance, the board is usually composed of responsible upper-class citizens well known in the community; if governmental, it will probably be under the jurisdiction of an official agency or a selected group of public officials. In the instance of hospitals owned by religious orders, church organizations, unions, or doctors, the governing bodies represent the respective constituencies.

Directly under the governing body, according to the organization chart, is the administrator or director of the hospital who receives his authority from it. Formerly the position tended to be filled by a physician if the hospital were large and secular, by a nurse if it were small, and by a nun (generally a nurse) or clergyman if it were sectarian. In recent years, however, men trained in hospital or sometimes in business administration increasingly are filling this post or are serving as consultants to administrators. Except in very small institutions, the administrator usually has assistants ranging in number from one to five or six to whom he delegates responsibility and authority for carrying out designated functions. As a result of the experience gained in these positions, it is relatively easy for assistant administrators to move rather quickly into more responsible positions elsewhere. Some are beginning to see, however, that they can make a career for themselves in specialized work on the assistant level.

Below the administrator and his assistants, organization-wise, are all the services of the hospital that function under his general direction or at least under his supervision in budgetary matters. Communication moves between him, or an assistant to whom he has delegated the responsibility, and the head of each of these services. Only the medical service is independent of the office of the hospital administrator; the medical director reports to the board of trustees. Open channels of informal communication exist, however, between the medical service and the administrator, and the house staff come under his jurisdiction in other than strictly medical matters.

As an exception to this predominant pattern of organization, the Veterans Administration with its vast system of some 170 hospitals has provided for two administrators of coordinate importance. One is a hospital director, until recently called "manager," who is generally but not always a physician. He is in charge of running the hospital as a social institution with the aid of an assistant director. The other, always a physician, is the chief of staff with responsibility for overall direction not only of the medical program, but the programs of all the "paramedical" groups giving direct attention to patients. Since the position of chief of staff is an essential unit in the hospital's formal structure and since part-time as well as full-time physicians come under its jurisdiction, the medical staff of these hospitals has been integrated within the organization as is not the case in most general hospitals.

Except for the medical and nursing services, the accompanying diagram does not do more than name those services that would probably be found in a teaching hospital of this size. In some institutions, two or more of the functions listed here as separate services might be combined; in others, further subdivision has occurred, or totally new services have been added. A few of the services like maintenance, laundry, and dietary will consist of large numbers of employees; those like pharmacy, occupational therapy, or social service will at best consist of a mere handful of staff members. Although clinical psychology has been noted on the diagram, many general hospitals, even of the teaching variety, do not yet have a single clinical psychologist who is a regular member of the hospital staff.

Regardless of the size of the services, each has a head and the larger ones are arranged in bureaucratic fashion to represent various levels of responsibility and authority. Since services not concerned with direct patient care fall largely outside the scope of this monograph, no attempt has been made to portray their formal structure. The structure of the medical and nursing services has, however, been represented roughly on the accompanying chart. The other professions serving patients are organized in a similar fashion but because of their generally limited size the chain of command tends to be relatively short and relations more informal.

Nursing as an Arm of Hospital Administration

Note has already been made of the fact that the medical service is organized and operates largely outside hospital administration. Because the implications of this fact will be discussed presently, nothing further need be said here. Attention must be given to the nursing service, however, since it constitutes the right arm of the hospital administrator (or "both hands," according to one administrator) in his responsibility for the patient areas of the institution. The floors on which the patients' beds are located, the operating, delivery, recovery, and emergency rooms, and the central supply service are places where ability to observe the condition of patients, exercise judgment about what needs to be done, and maintain the necessary asepsis are of vital importance. So important are these functions that responsibility for them must be vested in trained persons. These persons, it is generally believed, should be answerable to the administration of the hospital through the director of nursing service, who is often represented on the organization chart as one of the assistant hospital administrators.

To minimize risk, for example, hospitals require that every order for medication be checked by a nurse before administering it; she even has the right to refuse to give a medication. (The common law, moreover, may find the nurse liable if she injures a patient through administering a drug that has been incorrectly prescribed.) Generally an error in writing an order is only a slip of the pen, but sometimes it results from the physician's having forgotten a complicating condition. Under such circumstances the nurse must be prepared to hold her ground, as in the instance where a nurse raised the question of a particular drug by telephone and the doctor replied that the order was correct. She then reported to the nursing supervisor that a drug had been ordered that would be exceedingly dangerous for the diabetic patient. The supervisor immediately called on the physician in person, and recalled to him the diabetes that the nurse had not mentioned because she assumed he remembered it. The doctor was so alarmed over his serious error that he went on the "dead run" to the ward to make sure that everything was all right.

As another example, hospitals deem it a primary obligation to protect patients (and also staff and visitors) from infections wherever possible. Hence nurses are charged with responsibility for asepsis not only on the patient floors and in the central supply service, but particularly in the operating, recovery, and delivery rooms.[1] Scrub nurses are expected to watch the surgeons to make sure that they do not contaminate "clean" areas. Persons may enter these special units only under prescribed rules that are enforced by the nursing supervisor. In some hospitals it is her function to teach sterile technique to medical as well as to nursing students when they first come to the operating rooms.

In institutions that are fortunate enough to have a complete house staff, many tasks are performed by these young physicians who are also under the jurisdiction of the hospital administrator, for which nurses assume complete responsibility elsewhere. What complicates this situation is the frequent lack of clarity in lines of responsibility between residents and nurses. Even patients' physical needs may be neglected because each professional group has left a particular matter to the other without thinking to mention it. Practices vary greatly from hospital to hospital, moreover, and hence unless new staff members are immediately oriented to the rules of the institution, difficulties will be compounded.

More important than any confusion about who is to perform certain functions is the fact that nurses are often charged with responsibility for various undertakings without adequate authority for carrying out that responsibility. Unless the hospital administrator is in an exceptionally strong position and gives nursing service full support, many individual nurses find themselves caught in situations, as will be seen shortly, that are damaging to their morale if not to patient care.

In addition to largely running the patient areas as representatives of hospital administration, nurses must also carry out doctors' orders, give nursing care, and coordinate the plans for total patient care. Another function that occupies the time and

---

[1] Aseptic techniques are often initially worked out and instituted by an "infection committee" composed of persons with highly specialized knowledge. For a description of how physicians are informed about procedures on the patient floors of one hospital, see Mrs. Marion Foster's "A Positive Approach to Medical Asepsis" in *American Journal of Nursing*, vol. 62, April, 1962, pp. 76–77.

attention of perhaps a considerable number of persons in the nursing service, as well as the board of trustees that must concern itself with the financial aspects, is a school of nursing. Some 1,100 hospitals still operate such schools. Whether there be a school or not, in-service training of aides, orientation of practical and staff nurses, and continuing education in clinical procedures are receiving progressively larger attention.

Because of all these activities nursing is by far the largest of the services in every general hospital. (About half of the total budget is allocated to it.) The necessary introduction in the past two decades of so many categories of personnel into its structure makes the chain of command exceptionally long and cumbersome. To facilitate vertical communication and increase overall direction, supervisors, who may also be clinical nursing instructors, are appointed in all large hospitals to posts intermediate between the director and the head nurses.

At present in a few places "lay managers" of patient areas are being introduced to relieve head nurses and supervisors of those aspects of administration, above the competence of most secretaries, that do not require specific medical and nursing knowledge and judgment. Such persons of necessity now have to be initiated into their new jobs by nurses, and in some hospitals they are continuing to work under the supervision of the nursing service. Thus still another category is introduced into its hierarchy. In other hospitals it is believed that lay managers should be assigned to, and directed by, hospital administration, and that these managers should assume the task as soon as possible of training more personnel for the work.

As the hospital's nursing service has grown in size and is coming to realize how central a position of importance it holds, some nurses have begun to advocate that this service should be more largely self-directing, as is the medical service, and not under the jurisdiction of the hospital administrator. Hence they are recommending that there be an executive director at the head of any large teaching hospital to whom the medical director, nursing director, and hospital administrator would each answer independently. Whether such action will finally result in more than a few experimentally minded institutions remains to be seen. The suggestion is one of many for drastic reorganization of the formal structure of the hospital.

Patients and the Organization Chart

On the chart reference appears to *places* where patients have beds, deliver their babies, and undergo treatment including surgical intervention. But there is no reference whatsoever to patients themselves. The location on the diagram of these patient units suggests the distance that separates them from the chief sources of authority. Consequently, it would appear obvious, if this sample chart portrays relationships with any considerable validity, that patients are likely to have their most frequent contacts with medical and nursing staffs on the lower hierarchical levels. Directives flow down the long vertical lines of authority in the form of written and oral orders, rules, and prescribed procedures, while communication in an upward direction tends to move slowly, if not with great uncertainty. Therefore, unless patients have a personal physician or a strong and interested nursing supervisor to intercede for them, they are likely to find themselves, as subsequent illustrations will indicate, unable to make effective requests.

Actually patients are not considered to be within the organizational structure of the hospital for acute disease, or even within the social system that stems from the formal and informal structure. They are rather, as Dr. Wessen suggests, "a reference group in the midst of which the personnel operate, which they serve, and toward which they orient many of their actions and attitudes."[1] They are viewed by the staff much as transient guests, who do not understand the social system of the hospital or the therapeutic program that has been designed for their benefit. Like all good guests, they are expected to accede with the best possible grace to the plans made for them, and not to wear out their welcome if it can possibly be avoided. Many of the stresses about which patients complain stem, we believe, from the reluctance of the hospital to permit them to feel that they are a part of it.

[1] Wessen, Albert F., "Hospital Ideology and Communication Between Ward Personnel" in *Patients, Physicians and Illness*, edited by E. Gartly Jaco. The Free Press, New York, 1958, p. 449.

WHAT THE ORGANIZATION CHART FAILS TO DESCRIBE

The sample chart reproduced on page 58 appears clear and understandable. Anyone who accepts it, however, as a realistic picture of how social interaction actually operates in a hospital would be seriously misled.[1] It is a pattern appropriated in recent years from industrial and business organizations, which persons trained in hospital administration have found useful in attempting to describe and systematize rules and relationships for carrying out the management tasks of the institution. It does not record the effect of the historical development of the medical profession upon current practices. Hence it must be viewed as only a partial record of the formal structure of the general hospital.

The Competing Chain of Command

What the organization chart completely fails to describe is the other chain of command stemming from the medical director, as it affects many of the services of the hospital. The very fact that there are two competing hierarchies frequently results in weakening the nature of the social structure as portrayed on the chart and in causing great confusion. We have already noted that, except for house staff, physicians stand outside the system of organization of most general hospitals other than those operated by certain official agencies or departments.

The medical service works within its own pattern of rules and relationships, which is also bureaucratically ordered.[2] In addition, it exercises much authority over all the other professionally and technically trained groups that are directly concerned with patient care. Had this latter fact been portrayed on the organization chart, a horizontal line representing the entire medical service, except for students, would have cut across each service

[1] For a sociological discussion of four different kinds of organizational control in voluntary hospitals, see Perrow, Charles, "The Analysis of Goals in Complex Organizations," *American Sociological Review*, vol. 26, December, 1961, pp. 857–861.

[2] Physicians frequently make reference to a medical "team." Perhaps nothing reveals more clearly how little this term corresponds to what social scientists mean by "team" than the way in which the members of a medical team tend to group themselves on ward rounds. Where a doctor stands in relation to the "chief" and the patient generally suggests his rank in the hierarchical structure. When physicians on all levels are present, medical students are likely to be so far removed from the scene of action that they can see scarcely more than the back of the heads of the young doctors.

engaged in therapeutic functions. Such a line would indicate that communication is not confined to that between the medical director and the head of a particular service; theoretically any physician can initiate task-oriented communication, if he so desires, with any member of a service involved in attention to patients under his supervision.

In the evolutionary development of medicine and the health services, physicians long preceded other professional groups. Thanks to that fact, plus the extended academic and professional preparation required for practice and the degree of responsibility assumed by doctors and also legally ascribed to them, the medical profession has had a distinctive advantage. That advantage has been further accentuated by the relatively favored socioeconomic level from which doctors have been recruited, and the "charismatic" power with which society has endowed them. As a consequence of all these factors, physicians have had and continue to have the greatest authority, the highest status, and the largest prestige of any group within the hospital. Hence the medical service is able to extend its command directly over many of the services, and often, but more indirectly, over the hospital administrator.

Aside from their authoritative position in connection with the diagnosis and treatment of disease, however, the relative influence of doctors in the hospital has been diminishing.[1] The growth in the size of hospitals and the complexity of medicine have required that many new service and maintenance departments be created with which physicians concern themselves scarcely at all. By necessity if not by preference, doctors are delegating large numbers of functions, as has been noted, to an expanding number of other groups. These groups are rapidly moving toward professional skill and proficiency, and are beginning to insist that their role in the therapeutic process be enlarged. Frequently they receive considerable assistance in this effort from hospital administration.

The very fact, moreover, that only the house staff is integrated within the social system puts the medical service at some disad-

[1] See Robert N. Wilson's "The Physician's Changing Hospital Role," *Human Organization*, vol. 18, Winter, 1959–1960, pp. 177–183.

vantage. Almost everyone else works on a salaried and generally full-time basis, and hence the hospital is his work-world. The struggle that physicians have made to keep from coming under the jurisdiction of lay administration, although largely successful, results in their being excluded from many of the vital and satisfying aspects of that world. As "volunteers" to whom the hospital has accorded the privileges of membership in its medical staff,[1] they have relative independence; but like volunteers generally, they are cut off from much of the informal group life of the full-time workers that might make relationships between them and other personnel warmer and more comfortable. Quite as importantly, they are cut off from, or fail to interest themselves in, interdisciplinary meetings where plans are made and decisions taken in which they should participate or about which they at least need to inform themselves.

The Dual Value System

The two systems of authority and responsibility that characterize the average general hospital both reflect and exacerbate the duality of values that exists within it. Part of the staff considers that service to the patient is the paramount institutional objective; another part of the staff is concerned with economic and maintenance problems that determine to a considerable degree the quantity and quality of that service. Persons in the first group are frequently "impatient with, or stoutly ignore, administrative contingencies that appear to limit service to patients or that deflect their occupational goals."[2]

The second group see themselves involved in the important question of how to allocate funds that are never sufficient to meet seemingly unlimited wants, how to keep the several services staffed adequately to permit efficient service, and how to maintain a physical plant suitable to the changing demands of medical practice and community mores. This group conse-

[1] Wessen, Albert F., "Hospital Ideology and Communication Between Ward Personnel" in *Patients, Physicians and Illness*, edited by E. Gartly Jaco, p. 449.

[2] Smith, Harvey L., "The Major Aims and Organizational Characteristics of Mental Hospitals" in *The Patient and the Mental Hospital*, edited by Greenblatt, Levinson, and Williams. The Free Press, New York, 1957, p. 5.

quently find representatives of the first interest often very unreasonable. To use Dr. Smith's expressive comment, "It is small wonder, therefore, that hospitals seem to have a built-in sense of outrage."[1]

One hierarchical system is difficult to administer. Two such competing systems can scarcely fail to promote uncertainty, insecurity, friction, and the desire of each to advance its own ends. They seem to promote these undesirable characteristics more readily than they create the desire for careful examination of whether a better social system could be devised.[2] This kind of examination is retarded for several reasons. As yet very few non-medical hospital administrators are being trained broadly enough or have professional status sufficiently high to cope with such a knotty problem. In the face of the growing complexity of the hospital, medical staffs may exhibit more confusion, resistance, or indifference than helpful leadership. The several newer health professions are still unable clearly to define or defend their roles within the expanded system; and only now are general hospitals, unlike psychiatric institutions, taking the first steps toward having social science studies made of their social structure and how it actually operates.

PRACTICAL CONSEQUENCES OF THE EVOLUTIONARY PROCESS

Let us turn from these generalizations to two very simple situations that may be assumed to have their counterpart in all large hospitals where face-to-face contacts between the various professional groups are relatively infrequent or formal and often strained. Social situations have been chosen that deal with direct patient care, since they illustrate the consequences for sick persons of lack of clarity in roles. They also illustrate other conse-

[1] *Ibid.*

[2] For reports of research concerning status relations in one general and ten tuberculosis hospitals and the effect of those relations upon job satisfaction and performance, see *Measurement of Status Relations in a Hospital* by L. Edna Rogers; *Social Stratification and Personnel Turnover in the Hospital* by Ivar Oxaal; and *Stratification, Alienation, and the Hospital Setting* by John W. Evans. The first of these monographs was published in 1959 and the other two in 1960 by the Engineering Experiment Station, Ohio State University. See also Melvin Seeman and John W. Evans' "Stratification and Hospital Care" published in the February and April, 1961, issues of the *American Sociological Review.*

quences, which will shortly be discussed, that appear to be the direct outgrowth of the hierarchical structure. In the first incident presented there is inadequate definition of how authority should be shared between doctors on two levels, and what the responsibility of a nurse in a supervisory position should be to the patient and each of the doctors.

A patient who had been admitted to the private service of a voluntary hospital with hepatitis was told by the assistant head nurse on the morning following admission that she was to be taken for a chest x-ray. She said there must have been some mistake, inasmuch as she had only recently had a complete examination in her internist's office. The nurse replied that the x-ray had been ordered. Since the patient was almost certain that it had been ordered by the resident as a routine procedure and without consulting the attending physician, she suggested that the latter be asked for advice. The nurse, instead, politely but firmly talked the patient into having the x-ray as well as an electrocardiogram that had also been ordered. The patient consented because she wanted to be a "good guest," and because the nurse was in one of those frequent and difficult situations of finding herself caught between the resident's written order and the possible intent of the "attending." As a consequence the patient had an unnecessary dose of x-ray, and the Blue Cross fund received a large bill for two procedures that the internist promptly said, when he made his next call, he had not ordered and would not have recommended. He said, furthermore, that upon the patient's arrival, he had been about to note on the chart that no procedures were to be ordered without his approval. He had refrained because such notes "create tension in interpersonal relations," when the resident assumes that he is responsible for the care of the patients on the floor.

The second illustration is concerned with that extremely important question of who is to provide the patient, before he leaves the hospital, with the necessary counseling about what he may safely do or not do, and how he can best care for and adjust to a physical disability. Although nurses are increasingly being trained to conduct such counseling, it is often fortuitous whether the patient will receive the help he needs either from doctor or nurse. With ward patients nurses frequently carry on extensive and valuable counseling on the assumption that physicians are too busy. On the private floors of many institutions, however, they do not "teach" patients, because, to use their frequent expression, "the doctors would not like it."

The supervisor of a fine private pavilion made such a remark categorically to the writer. Some weeks later when she had forgotten her earlier statement, she related the following incident. An elderly man was to be discharged on crutches at noon on a particular day. Late in the morning it was discovered that he was apprehensive about returning to his apartment, lest he should be unable to get to the toilet unassisted. Quickly the nurses rearranged the furniture of the hospital room to resemble his room at home. Then a demonstration was given him of exactly how he could get out of his bed or chair and through the narrow bathroom door; he was asked to "return" the demonstration.

In commenting on this occurrence, the supervisor said the man had been taught in the physical therapy department to use crutches fairly well, but he was uneasy about handling them in difficult situations. Because of this fact and probable arteriosclerosis that made learning slow for him, she was sure he should have had practice sessions for several days before he was discharged. "And to think," she concluded, "we caught this problem only at eleven o'clock on the day he was to go home, and could not give him adequate preparation!" *Not a single reference did she make to the fact that it was inappropriate for nurses to do teaching on private floors.*

To persons accustomed to considerable autonomy and unacquainted with the hierarchical structure of the hospital, a relatively simple solution to such questions as those raised by the two illustrations comes immediately to mind. The failure, they would say, lies in communication. Why don't doctors and nurses discuss with each other what patients need, and decide how duties are to be allocated in order that such unfortunate occurrences may be minimized? Inadequate communication, not only between physicians and nurses but between all the various categories of staff, represents a critical problem for the hospital—so critical that it will be discussed in greater detail later. Here, however, we wish to emphasize other aspects of the social system, suggested by these illustrations, that are perhaps not so immediately obvious. They will be designated as multiple subordination,[1] and the conflict between dependency and authority.

[1] This term was taken from Dr. Jules Henry's article referred to earlier in the chapter, in which he explores in detail the consequences of "functional organization" in a psychiatric hospital.

1. Multiple Subordination

Because patients need to have so many different things done for them, the functional method that was described in the Introduction has developed as the seemingly most natural way of getting those things done. It leads, however, to overlap and multiplication of frequently contradictory orders. Since the personnel engaged to perform the functions are on many different levels of training and ability to exercise judgment, the hospital feels obliged to attempt to reduce randomness and minimize risk. Hence everyone in the upper echelons is likely to be concerned lest tasks are not being performed as he thinks they should be. As a result persons from these echelons "exercise anxious surveillance," to quote Dr. Henry's phrase, over persons below them.

The consequence is a system of multiple subordination in which an intern graduated from one of the best medical schools in the United States can, for example, be given orders by junior and senior residents, a clinical professor, or the chief of the service. He will receive many orders in the form of rules or directives from hospital administration, and the head nurse, as representative of the administration for a designated patient area, will tell him what he may or may not do concerning the use of that area. If a young doctor, who belongs to the most favored health profession, finds himself in such a position of multiple subordination, the situation is likely to be far more difficult for those other groups that give direct patient care.

In spite of this anxious surveillance there is frequently lack of clarity about spheres of activity and allocation of duties. Hence a worker may improvise his own theories as to his functions, while others improvise theories about what his functions are. Thus "a guessing game" develops and is eagerly pursued by both the functionary and those on whom he impinges. "Often the two guess at cross purposes. Out of vagueness of definition of function and multiplicity of signals there grow hostility, secrecy, conflicts over personal loyalties, and feelings of betrayal."[1] When hospitals attempt to reduce such ambiguities and conflicts and minimize risk, they sometimes only make patient care more in-

---

[1] Henry, Jules, "The Formal Social Structure of a Psychiatric Hospital," *Psychiatry*, vol. 17, May, 1954, p. 151.

adequate because they rely upon further rules to achieve their ends. These rules, presented in the form of written procedures with which staff are expected to familiarize themselves, can be so detailed that they almost deny the use of common sense even to qualified persons.

> One hospital, for instance, that was exceptionally fortunate in the educational background of its nurses had ruled that *no* medication (not simply narcotics and other dangerous drugs) should be given without a doctor's order. One evening an attending physician had himself admitted to that hospital as a patient because he had injured his back in lifting a man in cardiac failure out of a taxi. When the nurse came into his room, he told her that he had sedatives in his doctor's bag but that he would like her to bring him a laxative. She said she could not get it without an order. Said he, "But I am giving you an order." That was not permitted because his role had changed from physician to patient. He inquired who was on duty that evening to issue the order; it proved to be the intern working under his supervision. He picked up the bedside telephone and was about to call the intern when the nurse suddenly realized how ridiculous the situation was. "Put down that telephone," said she hastily as she went out to get the requested laxative.

2. The Conflict Between Dependency and Authority

Dependency upon rules and orders rather than upon one's own judgment is obviously required of many persons in numerous situations. This dependency, which is the product of the hierarchical structure and the functional division of labor, fosters psychological dependency. Such a state of affairs, Dr. Argyris reminds us in his discussion of organizations, makes "the individuals *dependent* upon, *passive* toward, and *subordinate* to the leader. As a result the individuals have *little control* over their working environment."[1]

In the instance of the nurse who talked the patient into going to the x-ray department, it is reasonable to assume that she had already succumbed to some degree of psychological dependency. Had she been asked whether she thought she had an obligation to represent her patient's interests, she would undoubtedly have replied in the affirmative. Yet in actuality she chose to neglect a

[1] Argyris, Chris, *Personality and Organization: The Conflict Between System and the Individual.* Harper and Bros., New York, 1957, p. 60.

patient's reasonable request in order to meet the expectations of the resident. Furthermore, she probably chose to carry out the resident's order rather than consult the senior internist, because she had to maintain more continuous relations with the former than with his superior and she did not intend to get into any conflict that could be avoided.

The second illustration of the elderly man's anxiety about using his crutches suggests that the grossly overworked phrase, "the doctors would not like it," may often be a rationalization for not "sticking one's neck out," even when it is apparent that a particular patient needs guidance that can be expertly given. That very rationalization can, however, be forgotten under favorable circumstances such as the support provided by a high-ranking nurse supervisor.

Anyone who has had a chance to observe nursing students from some of the collegiate schools, which encourage individual development, is often impressed by their keen desire to do whatever they can for patients. Sometimes they are able to maintain themselves as representatives of patients' interests to a remarkable degree even in tension-producing situations. If they later find themselves, however, employees within the rigid social system of many a large hospital, they are likely to regress into dependency rather than progress toward greater independence and autonomy. They may continue to believe that they are serving their patients; they may place great emphasis on the fact that they are professional persons. Yet, in reality, they may not know exactly who they are or what their attitudes and role should be.

Nursing service, as it exists in a considerable proportion of hospitals, has been unable to keep pace with nursing education, which is evolving within a relatively freer environment. As a result, some educational leaders have been heard to say that "what nursing service needs is a revolution." The writer is inclined to agree that action scarcely short of a revolution would be highly salutary in many places. It would be futile to assume, however, that persons suffering from such psychological dependency as the social system of the hospital induces, are likely to have the ego strength necessary to embark upon action of a very threatening nature. Were they women of great independence of spirit, they could probably achieve marked change in spite of their lesser authority when compared with that of physicians. They have two potent assets at their disposal: as already noted, they constitute by far the largest group that provides direct patient care; even more importantly, they are indispensable to the hospital. The vice president of a medical center, who was himself a physician, once remarked "Much as we should hate to do it, we could get along without doctors, and still do a great deal to help patients. But one cannot run hospitals without nurses."

Emphasis has been placed upon nurses because of their central position in patient care. It should not be assumed, however, that the other "paramedical" professions escape the handicap of multiple subordination. The hierarchical system does not permit them the freedom or the recognition that they desire, and that their professional training and experience frequently lead them to believe they merit. Generally they have rather clear-cut role expectations; when these expectations are not satisfied, they may suffer a sense of acute role deprivation.

Psychology has long pointed to the fact that when expectations are not met, rationalizations are easily found whereby an individual is able to explain why he did not have the needed opportunity or failed to accomplish as much as he could have under other circumstances. Thus he absolves himself from responsibility. If an aide, for instance, is reminded that his work leaves something to be desired, he can assure himself and perhaps others that he has too much to do, or his supervisor did not give him adequate directions, or the place is too "lousy" to merit his interest. What are valid reasons and what are rationalizations may be difficult to determine objectively.

To blame persons in positions of authority for one's dissatisfactions or shortcomings is very popular. It is much easier than blaming the complexities of a social system, particularly since almost everyone has been conditioned to think of persons rather than organizational patterns as causative agents. Staff members on the lower levels are likely to be resentful toward those who exercise direct authority over them; professional persons in each category of staff are likely to have ambivalent feelings toward the head of their particular department or the hospital administrator. The chief resentment among professional personnel, however, tends to be directed toward the physicians because each group identifies itself with them in its aspirations, but at the same time dislikes the power that they exercise.

They are not resented in their healing role per se, and as individuals they are usually respected, admired, and liked. Much of the resentment may be on the unconscious level. Many persons would deny having anything but respect for physicians, but the fact that some of them always show doctors a shade too much respect suggests subservience that can quickly turn into hostility. Others are so dependent upon the doctor for support that while he continues to give the help they need, he represents strength, reliability, and generosity. Let him withdraw that help and they may experience great bitterness.

A sample of incidents repeated over and again in hospitals will illustrate how closely related to one another authority and dependency or resentment may be, and how doctors who want to be cooperative may unwittingly increase friction or dependency.

On Monday morning a head nurse comes on duty to discover that her floor has had so many incontinent patients over the weekend that the generous supply of clean linen has been exhausted. Reluctantly she telephones the head of the laundry service to inquire if she can have more sheets. The respondent tells her with some asperity that she ought to know that she cannot be supplied on Monday when the laundry has been closed for two days.

Later the resident arrives to make his medical rounds. The head nurse apologizes for the condition of beds without fresh sheets, and says it will be difficult to get along until laundry is delivered the next morning. "Well, I guess if you need linen you can have it," he replies, reaching for the telephone. To the head of the laundry service he says pleasantly but incisively, "This is Dr. ——— speaking. We need clean linen on D4 and I should like you to get some right over here." "Yes, Doctor," answers an obedient voice. The laundry cart arrives.

The head nurse may react to this situation in one of two ways. She may feel grateful to the resident not only for helping her get what she needs at the moment, but for "running interference" with that "very unpleasant person" in the laundry (who is probably beset with several other requests on Monday morning). This is the road to dependency, not to conscious resentment. Or she may realize that a doctor who wanted to be helpful, has unthinkingly trespassed upon an area of responsibility completely hers, and hence has perhaps weakened her authority in dealing with the laundry service.

Here is the dilemma. Out of hundreds of situations as seemingly small and unimportant as this one, dependency is likely to develop that is not good for the individual and often not good for the institution. Another possible alternative is the gradual development of resentment toward that profession that has the authority to direct and supervise all medical aspects of patient care, and frequently extends its authority well beyond the strictly medical aspects. Even when physicians limit themselves conscientiously to what is supposedly their own province, the very fact that they can write orders for other groups to carry out may be a continuing source of friction. Some members of the staff will be inclined to view the orders as inadequate to meet the particular patient's needs; others, as lacking in specificity; still others, as so specific that their own competence to exercise judgment is not recognized. Under such circumstances physicians may be made to bear the blame for the evils of "the system."

To a lesser degree hospital administrators may find themselves in much the same position. The higher the status of the particular administrator, the more exposed will he be to possible envy, criticism, or resentment unless he be fortunate enough to direct an institution able to meet the psychological needs of staff reasonably well. What spares the administrator from much potential hostility, which physicians who are on the wards are not spared, is the fact that large proportions of the personnel are completely separated from him and from an interest in overall organizational goals. Thus their hostility, if expressed, is directed toward those with whom they have closer contact.

The administrator of a large hospital works with his board of trustees, his assistants, and the heads of the departments. The several assistants are often in positions where they may serve as buffers between some of the departments and him. Thus he may be appreciably isolated from many of the daily tensions that ebb and flow throughout the hospital. Even when this is true, he will still, perhaps, have to face the problem of the essential loneliness of his position. Often such persons admit to how *alone* they feel.

They have no small group, unless they and their assistants form one, on which to depend for psychological support. Interestingly, their loneliness seems rarely to be perceived with sympathetic understanding by their staffs. Is this because it is difficult to be emotionally generous to persons "at the top"?

THE NEED FOR POSITIVE LEADERSHIP FROM PHYSICIANS

The foregoing analysis leads to the conclusion, well summarized in Jules Henry's statement, "that an organization having specific characteristics can, through repetitively creating particular situations for the personnel working within it, bring about stresses in interpersonal relations, so that many persons, regardless of their personalities, will experience similar tensions. Obviously these tensions will have different ultimate effects on different people." To these observations he adds the suggestion that in an institution that has poorly functioning personnel "an administrator might ask himself *first* whether the poor functioning might not be due to some underlying defect in the organizational structure. It is not possible to put a group of even basically well-integrated persons into a poorly conceived organization and expect them to function without much stress."[1]

Persons who have attempted to examine the formal and informal structure of large institutions seem agreed that bureaucratic or hierarchical forms of organization pose serious questions about how operational efficiency can be achieved, while the basic psychological needs of the staff are protected.[2] Answers to these questions as they apply to large hospitals are still few in number. Later we shall describe several likely solutions which, however small, point hopefully to the possibility of finding other and perhaps more comprehensive ones.

Short of solutions, however, a broader understanding of, and insight into, the meaning of the hospital's social structure, both for staff and for patients, would appear urgently indicated. At present the knowledge about that structure and the dynamics of how the resulting social system works are so meager that many

[1] "The Formal Social Structure of a Psychiatric Hospital," *Psychiatry*, vol. 17, May, 1954, p. 151.

[2] See the excerpt from John Medelman's story, "It's Been a Long Snow," which appears as Appendix 4.

daily occurrences are unnecessarily exacerbated. The next chapter dealing with communication will carry this analysis farther. Here, following the discussion of multiple subordination and the conflict between dependency and authority, may be an appropriate place to add an important footnote specifically about physicians.

Much of the hospital literature understandably places great responsibility on the administrator for seeking to effect change. We have seen, however, that physicians are the group with the largest authority in matters pertaining to direct patient care, and consequently their attitudes and social behavior are important determinants of the climate of the hospital. With the notable exception of psychiatrists and many other individual doctors, they most unfortunately appear to have less knowledge and understanding of the relationship between the social system and social interaction than several of the other health professions, including hospital administrators.

Medical schools are beginning to make appreciable progress in introducing their students to some of the implications of psychiatry and the behavioral sciences for medical practice. Physician-patient relationships may receive considerable attention.[1] In the rehabilitation of the mentally ill or physically disabled, students may have a chance to see the use of a greatly expanded and integrated therapeutic team. In very few places as yet, however, do schools appear to give direct and systematic orientation to the role of the doctor *vis-à-vis* the representatives of the other professional groups with whom he will probably have to work progressively throughout his medical career. Little reference is made to the profound changes that are occurring in these professions, or to the fact that such changes may require alterations in his attitudes and in how he conducts his interpersonal relations. Attention to the social structure of the general hospital is usually lacking, although that institution will provide one of his important work areas and will require countless adjustments to its system different from those required in his private office.

---

[1] Gordon, Ira J., Peter F. Regan III, and Samuel P. Martin, "Role-Playing as a Technique for Teaching Medical Students," *Journal of Medical Education*, vol. 35, August, 1960, pp. 781–785.

To no inconsiderable degree the tensions currently conspicuous in many hospitals revolve around the struggle of individuals and even entire groups of personnel to decrease their dependency, increase the recognition awarded them, and achieve higher status. Even the younger physicians, who reflect the somewhat broader training that medical schools have begun to provide, are not in so favorable a position as might be hoped for viewing these upheavals with intellectual objectivity and emotional understanding and for lending constructive assistance. Older physicians, who were conditioned to the smaller hospital where relations were easier and more informal, often find themselves confused by, and sometimes intolerant of, the seeming chaos. They remark on the fact that many of the staff "always seem to have a chip on their shoulders." Instead of trying to make careful examination of what is occurring and decide what their responsibility might be, such doctors tend to become defensive and sometimes appear as if their own status were being threatened.

At a meeting where the writer had been invited to discuss the social structure of the hospital, a physician asked why she wanted "to tear down the prestige of the medical profession." She was so surprised by his interpretation of what she had intended to convey that she could scarcely believe she had heard him correctly. She has discovered since then that there are likely to be a few doctors in any audience who, perhaps because of some deep-seated insecurity as well as unfamiliarity with social science language, mistake analysis for criticism of their profession. Such persons may do great damage in their home hospitals if they act as though they thought their "prestige" were at stake.

Does anyone really believe that prestige is something limited in amount, and that there is not enough to go around? If so, he will almost certainly attempt to grasp it for himself and the profession he represents, and will try to deny it to other groups. On the other hand, if he views prestige as a good medication capable of reducing some of the social pains, he may conclude that it ought to be dispensed therapeutically insofar as possible to everyone who works in the tension-laden setting of the hospital. Should he decide that he and his profession, who have benefited greatly from this medication, become dispensers of it to others, may he not discover later that doctors have actually increased their own prestige in the eyes of a grateful institution?

Positive leadership from the medical profession, as well as from hospital administration, in coming to grips with some of the liabilities of the hospital's social system is sadly needed and sorely wanted. In his talk on "The Rehabilitation of Chronic Patients in Hospitals," to which we referred at the end of Chapter 2, Small Work Groups, Dr. John Cumming showed how such leadership could be provided at certain focal points, and in ways that would help staff move toward more maturity and independence of judgment rather than dependency, and toward greatly increased interest in patient care. To achieve this end the physician must be willing to devote some little time to the undertaking and more importantly he must be able—lest he create resentment—to lay aside at least some of the symbols of authority and status.

The reader will recall Dr. Cumming's gentle prescription to the physician: that he develop informal acquaintanceship with nurses (or other categories of staff), that he cultivate an interest in *their* problems, that he finally suggest the desirability of small group meetings at which those problems relating to patients and the hospital social system could be discussed. A considerable number of psychiatrists have now demonstrated that, having divested themselves of the use of power as it is conventionally portrayed, they have had marked success in helping personnel to make more of an emotional commitment to patients. Simultaneously, their own prestige has frequently grown in the hospitals or agencies with which they have been associated, and often among their colleagues the country over who have found positive, realistic suggestions in their papers for the upgrading of patient care.

Chapter 4

COMMUNICATION AND COORDINATION OF PATIENT CARE

COMMUNICATION IS SERIOUSLY IMPEDED, we noted earlier, by the organizational structure of the hospital and its resulting social system. Here further attention must be given to this problem that every large hospital, like most complex industries and business enterprises, finds a very serious one. Communication is, in fact, of paramount importance since coordination of patient care depends upon it. When no fewer than twenty-three different occupational status groups can be counted on a typical ward or unit,[1] one gets some realization of the amount of communication needed and of how easily failure to achieve coordination of service can occur.

But factors other than the mere number of persons involved are significant, as everyone knows. Extensive study of the subject of communication, much of it based on careful experimental research, has resulted in distinguishing the characteristics of various factors that appear to be important determinants of the amount, nature, and success of communication in a given situation. The early part of this chapter, therefore, will be devoted to the question of how much communication occurs between the groups involved in direct patient care, and to causes that theoretically at least might explain its paucity.[2]

[1] Wessen, Albert F., "Hospital Ideology and Communication Between Ward Personnel" in *Patients, Physicians and Illness*, edited by E. Gartly Jaco. The Free Press, New York, 1958, pp. 449–450.

[2] For helpful discussion of communication, including suggestions for improvement, written expressly for administrators of large organizations generally, see Strauss and Sayles' *Personnel: The Human Problems of Management*, Prentice-Hall, Inc., Englewood Cliffs, N. J., 1960, pp. 195–216, 307–326, 382–385; Jay M. Jackson's "The Organization and Its Communication Problems" in *The Journal of Communications*, vol. 9, December, 1959, pp. 158–167; and D. K. Waugh's "Training for Effective Communication," a talk reproduced in this monograph as Appendix 5.

Then a representative incident will be described at considerable length, involving one patient and three departments of a general hospital, to indicate the difficulty of establishing communication and coordination sufficient to permit a relatively small but individualized service to be performed daily. Finally, illustrations will be given of efforts to help nurses, who carry major responsibility for coordination at the ward or patient floor level, develop easier communication with other professional staff.

WHY LATERAL COMMUNICATION IS IMPEDED

In the preceding chapter we posed, and sought to give partial answers to, the question of why physicians and nurses do not discuss together the needs of their individual patients and come to some conclusion about their respective roles in meeting those needs. Here, in these pages focused upon the subject of communication it should be possible to give additional answers; answers, moreover, that refer not only to verbal transactions between doctors and nurses but to lateral transactions among all the health professions involved.

As evidence of the amount of oral communication that actually occurred between physicians and nurses in one institution, we should like to refer to the observations made some years ago by Dr. Albert F. Wessen, a sociologist, of social interaction at the nursing stations of a semiprivate and a ward unit in a highly favored voluntary hospital of more than 500 beds.[1] According to his count, a doctor was three times as likely to speak to another doctor while he was in the unit as he was to a nurse; he almost never talked to any other member of the staff. The nurse was more than twice as likely to speak with another nurse as with other personnel; her in-group communication was almost seven times as frequent as was her conversation with physicians. The twenty-nine per cent of her social interaction that was chiefly with nonprofessional persons resulted in part from the supervision she exercised, were she a head nurse or a team leader; in

[1] "Hospital Ideology and Communication Between Ward Personnel," pp. 453–454.

part from her membership in the small work group, were she a staff nurse.

Certainly the amount of lateral communication may differ widely from one patient unit to another in the same hospital and from institution to institution. However, on the basis of her own unsystematic but frequent observations and those reported to her by acquaintances, the writer would conclude that these figures are broadly representative of existing conditions in hospitals for acute disease.

Observations, carefully designed and scrupulously carried out, need to be repeated in a variety of situations. Without such authoritative data many persons will almost certainly continue to discount the real seriousness of the problem because they will believe, as did one physician occupying a strategic position, that oral communication is much greater than suggested here. Or they will consider the written orders, procedures, rules, and directives an adequate, perhaps preferable, substitute. That particular physician, who had no illusions about the sufficiency of written communication, was so surprised when Dr. Wessen's figures were presented that he asked twice to have them repeated. Said he thoughtfully, he had no idea that such conditions existed; he proposed to do whatever he could to change them.

Information is even scantier concerning the amount of social interaction that physicians and nurses engage in with other professional groups, such as dietitians, social workers, physical and occupational therapists, pharmacists, or dentists, who contribute to patient care. The one exception is the head nurse or nursing supervisor. In the process of coordinating plans for the care of individual patients and administering the patient unit, she has occasion to make contacts, generally by telephone, with most departments in the hospital.

Still less seems to be known about lateral communication among those groups mentioned in the preceding paragraph who are scattered throughout the hospital and rarely meet on the patient floors. The psychiatric, rehabilitation, and perhaps pediatric services of some hospitals now have regular meetings of the members of a therapeutic team, which may bring together a considerable diversity of personnel. Otherwise, the oral communication that moves back and forth among the staff who are not at the bedside may make the conversation between doctors and nurses appear relatively abundant.

Inadequacy of Written Communication

Having set down these preliminary statements about a probable dearth of oral transactions, something must be said concerning the reasons for inadequacies in the extensive written communications on which large hospitals place great reliance. Then we shall be ready to return to the basic question of *why* oral communication is so limited.

Doctors' written orders are very brief and are generally confined to medications, diagnostic tests to be done, special diets to be requested, and physical treatments to be given. Sometimes they include a request for continued observation of a patient. *TLC* occurs frequently enough, although chiefly in pediatrics, for all nurses to know that it stands for "tender, loving care." On a few psychiatric units, at least, attempts are being made to prescribe the attitudes that the staff are to use with the individual patient, after they have had didactic and clinical teaching in the nature and application of those attitudes. In general, however, doctors' orders are concerned with procedures for the treatment of disease rather than with the care of the patient as a person. They rarely include directions that could be written only after complex psychological, social, and cultural factors had been taken into consideration through pooling the observations and suggestions of several people.

Even orders dealing with the customary procedures for the treatment of disease present many problems. For example, if "complete bed rest" can be interpreted in ten slightly different ways, the interpretation that the individual nurse makes may or may not conform to what the physician intended. This creates uncertainty for the person charged with responsibility, and possible detrimental effects for the patient.

When we turn to the written orders, rules, and directives issued by hospital administration and the heads of the several departments, we can only conclude that the degree of understanding and acceptance that will be given them is generally unpredictable. American culture in mid-twentieth century appears more intolerant of orders in any form than was probably true at the beginning of the century,[1] or is still true in some other countries. Unless people are very dependent upon authority or exceptionally free from emotional resistance to it, orders signed by top executives, particularly if frequent, are likely to set up strong feelings of opposition.

Some years ago an administrator was finally selected for a particular hospital that needed to be raised to higher proficiency. The director of a neighboring institution was much interested in prospective developments. When the latter was asked his opinion six months later, about the choice of administrator, he replied, "I am afraid a bad mistake has been made." His only evidence for that conclusion, said he, was the large number of rulings being posted throughout the hospital signed by the administrator. He considered the practice almost worthless, generally pernicious, and likely to get the new executive off to a poor start. He questioned how many would remember the rulings even if they were read and understood. He assumed that some persons would be unconsciously resentful enough to sabotage their intent, if only by forgetting to examine them.

Written directives that hospitals distribute use language that is generally too difficult for those considerable segments of a large staff that have not had much education. It has been well said that most written communications, whether in business, industry, or hospitals, look as if they had been prepared by college people for college people. Even more important, however, than the language used is what the reader interprets the words to mean. Meaning is subjective. "It is affected by individual differences, attitudes, experiences, and the situation at the moment."[2] The communicator (or sender) of a message cannot give meaning to the receivers. He uses symbols that he hopes will transmit his meaning; what the receivers take from those symbols depends on

---

[1] "When I was a daughter, it was a crime to resist authority; when I became a mother, it had become a crime to assert it." (Peterson, Virgilia, *A Matter of Life and Death*, Atheneum Press, New York, 1961, p. 183.)

[2] This quotation, as well as some of the other generalizations about communication, appears in D. K. Waugh's talk, "Training for Effective Communication," reproduced as Appendix 5.

their own experiences and attitudes. Their interpretation may be so different from what the communicator intended that the latter sometimes wonders whether he or they are "nuts."

At best, barriers to common understanding are so great that they often produce inaccurate rumors, as well as distortions and breakdown in the attempts of large organizations to transmit information to their personnel. Messages transmitted in writing are viewed by students of communication as the least effective means of producing understanding. Only when the sender of the message has direct contact with the receiver can he hope to know what the latter hears and understands. Face-to-face inter-action is regarded, therefore, as far superior to written communi-cation; even it fails unless the communicator is prepared to adjust himself to the receiver by actively listening to "what is going on" and by showing interest and respect.

Hypotheses About the Nature of Oral Communication

References have been made throughout this monograph to the professional groups, increasing in number, that compose a sig-nificant proportion of the hospital's staff. It is now essential to take a closer look at these groups, since they determine to no insignificant degree the nature and amount of communication that concern patient care.

Every profession understandably prides itself upon the body of knowledge and the skills it has developed. It likes to think of them as unique, even though both knowledge and skills may overlap those of other groups in varying degrees. As part of their training, students not only learn a specialized vocabulary, they are almost unconsciously warped into the value system that the profession has evolved and that they will zealously guard. Most unfortunately, that specialized vocabulary and a value system that includes a large element of exclusiveness, immediately set up barriers to communication.

No profession wants to share too much of its hard won "stock in trade" with other professions, even though it must work in the closest contact with them to achieve a common purpose. (For the same reason it is reluctant to share even enough of its heritage with patients to permit them, whatever their educational background, to be other than guests in the general hospital.) This partially explains the comments overheard when members of one profession, often without factual basis for their statements, speak of the inadequate preparation or the lack of judgment or "maturity" of another group, as reasons for not wanting to include the latter in significant activities that they consider their province.

The perceptual distortions that result from the seeming need to minimize the role of other professional groups in order to maximize one's own, may be as exaggerated as the remark of the medical social worker who said that she did not know that nurses were interested in patients as individual persons. Or the categorical statement of a doctor that "nurses do not do research," in spite of the fact that research had been going on under his very eyes for almost a decade. Some members of all the health professions still appear to believe that medical social workers are trained only to attend to the economic problems and living arrangements of financially or socially disadvantaged patients; while physical and occupational therapists are primarily concerned with keeping patients occupied and helping to strengthen a few weak muscles.

It is as if the several professions preferred not to learn about each other's areas of competence, lest the knowledge be too threatening to them. The fact that many hospitals now operate only one large dining room where all categories of staff go for coffee and meals does relatively little to improve communication. The very seating arrangements tend to perpetuate cleavages between the groups.

The consequences for communication of these group-centered perceptions are greatly intensified by the formal structure of the hospital. An organizational pattern that fosters distinctive separateness among the professions, when combined with the tendency of those professions toward exclusiveness, is almost certain to reduce lateral communication. The very concentration of so much authority and status near the top of the structure, suggests that even the limited oral communications that occur between groups will be greatest there, thus leaving little social interaction at levels closest to the patients.

Moreover, although the formal structure appears to foster vertical communication within each group, much information that is needed may not get below or above the level of the supervisors. This may be true in spite of the fact that one of the chief functions of supervision is to facilitate messages moving both downward and upward.

Mary T. Grivest has reported, in her study of the attitudes of nurses toward their work in four selected hospitals, that:

> Supervisors feel they have no difficulty in communicating with management and are free to verbalize and make known their ideas and complaints.
>
> The head nurses with responsibilities for production indicate they are grossly uninformed about future planning and are not free to offer suggestions. This would imply, on the one hand, that lines to and from management are open, but that, on the other hand, communications travel only to and from the middle management level. Either this is intentional or the supervisory group does not or perhaps cannot transmit the information necessary.[1]

Thus far the discussion has centered around the professions and the formal structure of the hospital as inhibiting factors in communication among groups. We must now give attention to another factor, implicit in some of the previous references to status position, that obviously plays an important role within most organizations in determining the direction in which both horizontal and vertical communication tend to move. This factor has received less attention than it merits in its applicability to hospitals and its implications for patient care. We refer to the desire of personnel generally to have contact with those in more favored positions than their own.

Professor Jay M. Jackson's article, to which bibliographical reference was made at the beginning of the chapter, is devoted in large part to a discussion of this form of social behavior and the reasons for its existence and prevalence. Because his analysis is exceptionally clear and seems so relevant to hospitals, a résumé of it is presented here. We begin by quoting one paragraph of Dr. Jackson's summary of the results of a study of communication

---

[1] "A Personnel Inventory of Supervisors, Head Nurses, and Staff Nurses in Selected Hospitals," *Nursing Research*, vol. 7, June, 1958, p. 86.

patterns among all the personnel from the director to the janitor of a medium-sized government agency.

It was found that people communicated far more to members of their own sub-groups than to any other persons. They also preferred to be communicating to someone of higher status than themselves and tried to avoid having communication with those lower in status than themselves. The only exception to this tendency was when a person had supervisory responsibilities which removed his restraints against communicating with particular lower status persons. When people did communicate with others of the same status level in the organization, there was a strong tendency for them to select highly valued persons and to avoid those they thought were making little contribution.[1]

From the various kinds of evidence available, Dr. Jackson concluded that a hypothesis might be stated as follows: "In the pursuit of their work goals, people have [motivational] forces acting upon them to communicate with those who will help them to achieve their aims, and forces against communicating with those who will not assist, or may retard their accomplishment."[2] Higher status persons have the power to create either gratifying or depriving experiences for others. These experiences may be in the form of tangible decisions and rewards, or merely expressions of approval and confidence. Persons in lower status positions need reassurance concerning their superiors' attitudes, evaluations, and intentions toward them. Hence a second hypothesis might be formulated to suggest that people tend "to direct their communication toward those who can make them feel more secure and gratify their needs and away from those who threaten them, make them feel anxious, and generally provide unrewarding experiences."[3]

Dr. Jackson's third hypothesis, which is closely related to his first, is of particular interest psychologically. He assumes that "persons in an organization are always communicating," whether they are aware of it or not, "as if they were trying to improve their position." It is well known that many subordinates are

---

[1] "The Organization and Its Communication Problems," *The Journal of Communications*, vol. 9, December, 1959, p. 161.

[2] *Ibid.*

[3] *Ibid.*, p. 162.

reluctant to ask supervisors for needed help, lest the latter interpret this as an admission of inadequacy. "Superiors tend to delete from their communications to subordinates any reference to their own mistakes or errors of judgment."[1]

Since many members of a staff undoubtedly want to belong to a higher status group, talking upward may be a gratifying substitute for moving upward. Those who are attracted to membership in a particular group will be inclined to direct their communication to that group more extensively than will those who do not want to belong. If they are barred from belonging, they may increase their communication still further as if this were a substitute for actual membership.

As a final example of how communication is used to improve one's relative position, Dr. Jackson refers to a study of role relationships among three professional groups who work together in the mental health field: psychiatrists, clinical psychologists, and psychiatric social workers. The study demonstrated that the direction, amount, and content of their communication to one another could be predicted largely from two factors: their perception of the power of the other professions relative to their own, and how satisfied they were with their own power position compared to that of the other groups.

COMMUNICATION AND MEETING PATIENTS' NEEDS

We now turn to the immediate problem of communication in its implications for patient care and also for the motivation of workers that provide that care. From the foregoing generalizations it must be assumed that communication tends, first, to flow profession-wise or group-wise; it tends, second, either to be easily blocked by lateral barriers or to flow, unless supervisors change its direction, toward persons of higher status. Under such circumstances, how is it possible to get adequate information moving horizontally and vertically to the persons who need it for essential planning and coordinating of patient care? How is it possible, furthermore, to provide the motivation required by staff in positions less favored but nevertheless central to patient care, if they are to be willing to make any considerable commitment to their

[1] *Ibid.*, p. 163.

jobs? The remaining sections of this monograph will be largely devoted to attempted answers to these questions.

Before proceeding, however, let us look at an actual situation reported at some length by the patient involved. Unfortunately, we have only her perceptions, and many important facts about the communication that took place or did not take place across departmental and status lines, were not at her disposal. Nevertheless, the incident will serve to sensitize the reader to the difficulties inherent in coordinating the efforts of three departments and of persons on various status levels sufficiently to assure the patient of one small service not provided as part of the regular procedure.

On the morning after the patient had entered a well-known voluntary hospital, a dietitian came to discuss with her a food regime high in protein and sugar. At the end of the conference the dietitian inquired pleasantly but in a somewhat perfunctory way if there was anything the patient would like to suggest. The latter innocently said that she would like to have early morning coffee and prune juice.

During a previous stay in the same hospital a nurse had suggested the desirability of coffee and prune juice taken well before breakfast to counteract the effects upon digestion of large amounts of sedation. Every morning at seven o'clock an attractive tray had arrived with a pot of delicious, very hot coffee and a glass of prune juice set in a bowl of ice. The patient had discovered how effective was this prescription not only for the designated purpose but for relieving any slight morning depression.

Because of her earlier experience the patient assumed that coffee would be available to anyone who asked for it. Had she realized the difficulties she was about to provoke, she would not have made the request. The dietitian inquired when the coffee was wanted. At mention of seven o'clock she said, with an attempt to conceal the sharpness in her voice, that that would be impossible since the staff did not arrive until seven thirty and it took an hour to make coffee. The patient showed surprise, referred to how coffee had been served during an earlier hospitalization, and mentioned the fact that she had smelled coffee that very morning in the corridor just outside her door. The dietitian commented that the part of the private pavilion where the patient had had a room previously was provided with its own kitchen and staff, and hence could meet specific requests; if she had smelled coffee, the nurses had undoubtedly made it for themselves. (In fact, the kitchen used by the nursing staff was far down the corridor.)

Just then the patient's personal physician walked into the room. He listened, and as a psychiatricly oriented internist who recognizes the therapeutic value of positive action and individualized patient care, suggested that there certainly ought to be some solution. The dietitian inquired about powdered coffee, which the nurses could provide; the patient was willing to settle for that. Suddenly the physician said almost gaily that *he* had thought of something. He would bring a thermos bottle and the dietitian could arrange to have it filled each evening and put on the bedside table. A bottle of prune juice could be given to the head nurse to be kept in the refrigerator on the floor. In the mornings the nursing aide on duty would bring a glass of the juice and a cup and saucer. "That is all there is to it," he concluded. The dietitian apparently knew that that was not all there would be to it. She accepted the plan, but the expression that the patient caught on her face seemed to say that if anyone in a lesser position had made the suggestion, she would have firmly refused.

A charming, brightly colored thermos bottle promptly arrived and was put on the bedside table. It was not filled that evening, but the next morning a nursing aide appeared with powdered coffee and prune juice. During the forenoon the assistant head nurse came to see the patient three times, first to tell her that nursing and dietetics were working on a procedure, and then to report that she thought a solution to the problem was going to be found. The expenditure of energy and of time spent in telephoning must have been very large.

For three evenings a Negro girl of about eighteen arrived from the kitchen to get the thermos bottle. Her attitude was the perfect stereotype of what one might expect "kitchen help" to be like. She had probably had so disadvantaged a life emotionally, educationally, and economically that she acted as if she "didn't give a damn about anything." The contrast between her and the nursing aides on the floor, some of whom were remarkable women, was conspicuous indeed. She would seize the bottle and shortly afterward bring it back perhaps with coffee dripping down the outside. The patient would discover the following morning that the coffee was cold and too bitter to drink. Apparently the bottle had not been washed or heated with hot water and the coffee used had been made hours earlier.

When the girl from the kitchen had her two days off duty, no one came to get the thermos bottle. The patient had already decided that she could not drink the coffee. Hence, the failure of anyone to appear was important only because it demonstrated how difficult it is, with the hospital's complex staffing pattern, to guarantee sufficient communication to individualize even a small segment of patient care on a systematic basis.

Once or twice after the girl's return from her days off duty, she came with obvious annoyance to get the bottle. Nothing that the patient might say elicited a spark of interest. A generous tip would perhaps have provided better service, but it would also have raised several difficult questions. From the patient's point of view the minimum daily charge of $35 for a very modest private room seemed sufficient to permit a little individualized attention, provided pleasantly by persons who worked under favorable enough conditions so that pleasantness might be expected of them. On the other hand, she thought it likely that many of the persons connected with the food and maintenance services were very poorly paid. At the same time the hospital was struggling, probably without great success, against the system of patients' tipping employees.

Somewhat later the head nurse inquired how the coffee plan was working. When told that it had long since been written off, she said that she was going to see what could be done. The attending internist also inquired and suggested that he write a doctor's order, thereby almost guaranteeing that coffee would be served, regardless of its quality. The patient replied that she did not think the problem was a medical responsibility, and hence she concluded that she, nursing, and dietetics ought to see whether it could be solved without an order.

Two days after the head nurse's remark the girl suddenly reappeared to pick up the bottle. As she hastily reached for it on the bedside table, she brushed the patient's traveling clock with a wide sweep of her arm onto the floor. Ten minutes later she was back, accompanied by two other girls of her age from the kitchen, who stood wide-eyed in the doorway waiting to hear the reprimand that they certainly expected would follow. The patient felt too frustrated by the failure of her struggle, however, to mention the clock that lay broken under the bed. The girl was never seen again.

During all this time a nursing aide had continued to bring the prune juice with almost no lapses. If it failed to appear, the patient had only to ask for it over the "intercom" system. Finally, even the early morning prune juice came to be undependable because of the interference of medical procedures. One morning when it did not arrive and the patient asked for it, a voice replied, "You are fasting this morning until blood has been drawn."[1] Blood was taken, and the prune juice was brought with the breakfast, thereby supposedly decreasing its effectiveness. Because the senior internist had said that the blood tests had been completed, the patient was surprised to hear

[1] Hospitals interested in improving communication between staff and patients might profitably wipe out the word "fasting," which is commonly employed when a meal has to be omitted or delayed for medical reasons. It carries a connotation of punitiveness for many patients, and recalls Thomas Bell's perception of the hospital as so niggardly in its food service that he had a premonition he would "die hungry" in such a place. (*In the Midst of Life*, Atheneum Press, New York, 1961, p. 165.)

the same voice announce two days later, "You are fasting today." When the chief resident himself arrived to take more blood, the patient thought that this was an opportunity to make a request that might be helpful to her and perhaps to others, since he was the one who wrote most of the orders.

She asked him quietly if it would be possible, were he to order blood taken again, to have her or the nursing staff informed the night before. Her communication was obviously inadequate. The message that he seemed to receive was a complaint because the morning meal was either being delayed or canceled. He replied that breakfast would be served as soon as he had finished. When she explained that it was not a question of breakfast but of needing to request a cathartic at night if prune juice were not to be available the following morning, he showed no indication that the matter was of any importance. The patient could only conclude that an effort to coordinate procedures was unlikely, although constipation of bed patients is regarded as serious enough to warrant daily inquiries by the nursing staff, who are then expected to take action as indicated.

Although this case study appears to the writer to speak for itself, there are undoubtedly persons who might find the situation portrayed so inconsequential that they would ask, "Why all the fuss? Hospital staffs should give their time and attention to more important matters." Inherent in the comment is the supposition that when vital matters are at stake communication will function more adequately. Two exceptions must be made to these assumptions. First, much of a hospital's activity, for the great majority of the staff concerned with patient care, is composed of just such small and seemingly unimportant details. When these details are added together, however, they form a composite picture of therapeutic effectiveness or ineffectiveness, if "therapeutic" be used to indicate attempts to meet the needs of a patient-person. Second, the ability of a hospital to establish adequate channels of communication and to achieve coordination of effort can perhaps be better measured by these everyday occurrences than by the dramatic but unrepresentative emergencies that may be capable momentarily of calling upon cooperative, willing endeavor.

IMPROVING NURSES' SKILL IN COMMUNICATION

The preceding illustration is intended to suggest that many efforts of many kinds will have to be made before it becomes possible for members of different professions and status groups to focus action at the point of the patient's need without undue delay or stress. Many of these efforts will revolve around improvement in verbal communication. The next three chapters will be largely concerned with other facets of such efforts, including the use of nonverbal symbols that have meaning for staff or patients, and of undertakings that are not generally classified under the rubric of communication. Therefore we wish to focus attention in this concluding section upon two attempts to develop greater ease in verbal communication. The two incidents selected involve nurses, since they represent the channel most frequently used in transmitting messages regarding patient care.

In the first instance, better lateral communication by doctors rather than nurses was desired. However, the leader, himself a physician, did not know how to approach the problem directly, because he realized that the communication pattern to which physicians have been conditioned restricts the great majority to conversation with their own professional group. Hence a plan was made for helping nurses to *initiate* communication with doctors, in spite of the fact that clearly they would be in so vulnerable a position they would have to be supported. In the second case, an experiment was begun in reducing the relative inability of head nurses to be full participants in meetings of therapeutic teams where a highly developed word-skill was a prerequisite.

Although the voluntary hospital where the first undertaking occurred had well-qualified attending physicians and well-prepared nurses, many thought that patient care on the private floors might be improved. The basic difficulty lay in insufficient discussion by the "attendings" with the resident doctors and the nurses about what should be done for the patients. It was customary for a private physician to hurry to a floor, visit his patient or patients, write brief orders, and leave. Often he would not even see the resident because the latter might well be in a different part of the hospital at the moment. The head nurse did not accompany him, since twenty different doctors might come to the floor in a morning, several at the same time.

An internist who had had long and valuable experience in working closely with the nurses and house staff to the great benefit of his patients, decided, with the approval of the chief of service, to see whether some changes might be made through indirect means. After considerable planning with the director of nursing service and the supervisor of the private pavilion, he began holding weekly meetings with the nursing staff of one of the private floors. The appropriate house staff and attending doctors were cordially invited, but rarely appeared because they were "too busy." (Although this phrase unquestionably states a fact in many instances, clinicians cannot often be encouraged to attend meetings that extend across professional lines. They do, however, find time to attend clinical presentations in large numbers.)

The meetings focused for some weeks upon the problems that the nurses encountered. Many of their frustrations that they brought up for discussion revolved around poor arrangement and equipment of work areas, delays in receiving supplies, and so on. Some of these situations could be improved rather quickly. During this period the internist suggested to the chief of service the desirability of separating medical and surgical patients who had customarily been treated on the same floors in the private pavilion. When this rearrangement was introduced, it did much to bring the residents into easier contact with the attending doctors. It proved, however, to be less helpful to nursing. Because many more nurses prefer to work with surgical than with medical patients, the floors exclusively for medical cases began to have difficulty in maintaining their nursing quotas.

After the meetings had been going on for several months, it was decided to develop a schedule of questions about various aspects of patient care that could profitably be discussed with the attending physicians. When the schedule was ready, it was proposed that the nurse who had considerable contact with a particular patient should approach his private doctor while the latter was on the floor. She should introduce herself, and assure the physician that the nursing service wanted to give the best possible care to his patient, Mr. X. To make certain that they were giving full attention to the medical aspects of such care, the nursing service—so she was to comment— felt the need of obtaining his suggestions about what he thought might be done. If the physician responded by discussing the patient, talking about patient care in general, or any other subject that might lead to open channels of communication, the nurse was not to use the schedule. If the doctor proved unresponsive, however, the nurse was to ask him a specific question taken from the top of the list. She was then to proceed, if possible, from the more concrete and easy questions to the more complicated ones. With the carefully designed paper in her hand and the realization that the discussion group was standing behind her, it was thought that she might have adequate psychological support to hold her position when necessary.

Unfortunately, this experiment came to an end when only enough testing had been done to suggest promising results. It would appear sufficiently valuable to warrant trying in places where private physicians are so unaccustomed to discussion with other categories of personnel that staff resources cannot be fully utilized. For purposes of experimentation, various alterations could well be made in the plans for initiating communication and for providing support.

A technique that has proved of exceptional usefulness in preparing individuals to meet just such situations is role playing.[1] Nurses might profitably be given the opportunity, in role-playing sessions under the guidance of an experienced person, to react to the various kinds of probable responses until they felt ready to undertake the task with more self-confidence. Some of them might even come to look forward with interest to seeing how much success they could achieve.

The second incident occurred in a large new psychiatric hospital. It had been provided with such a wealth of facilities and professional personnel that it felt under considerable pressure to discharge patients as rapidly as possible. To achieve this goal it considered therapeutic teams for general planning of patient care and discussion of individual patients with particular social problems a major instrumentality. In the teams that were composed of psychiatrists, nurses, social workers, and clinical psychologists, the nurses seemed at a considerable disadvantage. Although they sometimes had more information about the patient than did the others or information of a different but perhaps equally important kind, they appeared unable to bring it within the frame of reference generally utilized in the meetings. On the surface it looked as if these other groups had a better word-skill. This could logically be attributed to a longer academic training or to similarities in their professional preparation that more nearly gave them like ways of organizing their perceptions and theories.

The hospital continued to believe that the head nurse was potentially an indispensable member of the therapeutic team. Consequently, a clinical psychologist who had had successful experience in group counseling, asked several head nurses and perhaps supervisors

[1] Harty, Margaret B., "Role Playing as a Teaching Technique," *Nursing Outlook*, vol. 9, September, 1961, pp. 563–564; Greenblatt, Milton, Richard H. York, and Esther Lucile Brown, *From Custodial to Therapeutic Patient Care in Mental Hospitals*, Russell Sage Foundation, New York, 1955, pp. 179–190.

if they would like to have him meet with them once a week to help them with more active participation. He suggested that when they felt comfortable enough with each other and with him, they invite one person of their choice who represented psychiatry, social work, or clinical psychology, to join the group. When they concluded that the newcomer was fully accepted, they were to select a second person from among the two remaining disciplines. Later they would choose the third person to complete the membership of a therapeutic team as constituted in that hospital.

The nurse who reported on this plan said that she and her colleagues had had a very fruitful experience and "had come a long way." "But," said she, "it has been a year since the weekly meetings began, and only now do we feel free enough to take the initiative and invite the first representative of another discipline to join us."

Because this interesting incident was presented at a large meeting where there was little opportunity to ask questions, we do not know what had occurred within the group. Nor do we know how much insight the nurses may have had into what was developing of psychological import. We think it reasonable to assume that they had established a close identification with the clinical psychologist who was the leader. Since the nursing profession does not have the degree of attention shown it by the medical profession that it craves, it tends to respond with exceptional warmth to representatives of other professions that clearly indicate an interest. Clinical psychologists are in a particularly favored position: they and nurses are noncompetitive, the majority are men, and they have skills in methods of research as well as in counseling that nurses want to cultivate and that psychologists sometimes share with marked generosity.

Through the probable identification with the clinical psychologist and their small-group relationships with each other, it may be assumed further that these nurses had gained ego strength that they greatly needed. And with that gain the ability to formulate and express ideas and opinions had been appreciably enlarged. It had taken the group an exceedingly long time, however, before they felt comfortable about inviting the representative of another discipline, even though he was to be of their own choosing and they worked in a hospital where the climate was generally permissive and supportive.

Around the very fact of such reluctance, important questions are involved that deserve careful examination. Answers to them would perhaps provide significant clues about *how* communication skills among nurses could best be fostered. Possible answers may be found both in social and in psychological factors. Sociologists might well interpret hesitancy in taking the initiative, particularly where physicians are concerned, to be the result of the conditioning of hospital schools of nursing that long placed excessive emphasis upon "respect shown doctors" and upon fitting unobtrusively into the social system. They might also consider it the product of the failure of all the professions, and particularly of the pivotal one, to demonstrate much concern for other groups. Finally, they would probably point to the disparaging attitude that professional persons trained in universities show toward hospital training with its element of apprenticeship, and toward higher degrees awarded by schools of education where emphasis has often been placed upon methodological questions at the expense of substantive knowledge.

Psychiatrists have advanced a very different theory when seeking to explain difficulties in nurse-physician communication. In their opinion many nurses unconsciously view the man physician in the role of father or husband to whom they should defer and with whom conflict should be reduced to a minimum. A deep-buried desire for dependency upon this role model may even be the motivation that attracts many girls to nursing initially. If there be validity in this theory, psychiatrists would consider that it constitutes a more serious problem to communication than does an inadequate word-skill per se or the factors to which the sociologists point.

Recently several behavioral scientists have attempted examination of the personality patterns of selected samples of nurses and nursing students,[1] that may throw further light on difficulties connected with communication. Regardless of the method and

[1] Mauksch, Hans O., "The Nurse: A Study in Role Perception," mimeographed abstract of doctoral dissertation submitted to the University of Chicago, April, 1960; Cleveland, Sidney E., "Personality Patterns Associated with the Professions of Dietitian and Nurse," *Journal of Health and Human Behavior*, vol. 2, Summer, 1961, pp. 113–124; Argyris, Chris, *Diagnosing Human Relations in Organizations*, Yale University, New Haven, 1956.

scope of each of these studies, the results point to a personality pattern characterized by high tolerance for passivity, and the conscious or unconscious need to receive succorance and to give nurturance. At the same time nurses appear to want clearly defined relations with those above and below them in the social structure, and they manifest a strong desire to avoid disapproval, blame, and failure. These characteristics are in sharp contrast to those expressed by the dietitians also examined in one of the studies, who were primarily concerned with prestige, status, and achievement, as were the hard-driving hospital administrators referred to earlier in this monograph.[1]

In connection with the incident cited above, it would be instructive to know to what extent the clinical psychologist who was the group leader took assumptions about unconscious motivations into consideration, and attempted to help the head nurses gain insight into their possible implications. Whatever the answer might be, skillful group counseling provides a potential opportunity for some unconscious motivations to be brought into consciousness where they can be looked at and analyzed,[2] and where the nurse (like other individuals) can gradually learn how to handle herself better when faced by persons who are symbols of authority or status. Group counseling might prove an important instrumentality whereby nurses could truly become representatives of the patient's interests as needed, even when they found themselves in conflict situations with physicians or other therapists.

So far as the sociological considerations mentioned above are concerned, time appears to be on the side of the nursing profession. Training is progressively being brought within higher education, increased attention is rapidly being given to the humanities and the social sciences, as well as the biological sciences, and larger numbers of nurses yearly are working not only for master's degrees and the doctor of education but for the degree of doctor of philosophy or science. Presently the content of clinical practice will be much enriched from the current ferment that is finding

[1] See p. 23.

[2] For a report of how a required course in Group Dynamics helped students in a School of Public Health to acquire self-awareness, see Dr. Irving S. Shapiro's "Can Human Relations Be Taught?" *Hospital Administration*, vol. 3, Fall, 1958, pp. 15–25.

expression in reexamination of basic assumptions, utilization of a wider body of knowledge about human behavior in health and sickness, and experimental undertakings in nurse-patient relationships. These trends should help to produce the self-confidence the profession needs. They should also help to win merited respect as the other health professions learn about them across the barriers to communication that occupational "ethnocentrism" creates. As that respect grows, it in turn should reinforce self-confidence and greatly encourage nurses to take their place as full participants in the therapeutic team.

Chapter 5

MOTIVATION

REVIEW OF EARLIER EXPERIMENTS IN MOTIVATION led psychologists to formulate the hypothesis, success = motivation $\times$ aptitude. Subsequent experiments appeared to demonstrate that motivation is even more important than had been assumed. Hence they have restated the hypothesis to read, success = motivation^2 $\times$ aptitude. Obviously, in any efforts to maximize the use of the human resources of the hospital in behalf of better patient care, the question of the level of staff motivation becomes one of paramount importance.

Hospitals are, of course, well aware of this fact but they have tended to rely predominantly upon the hope that improvement in salaries, fringe benefits, and physical working conditions would result in higher levels of motivation. Evidence seems to suggest that such emoluments may improve morale, but since everyone shares more or less equally in them, they provide no reward to the individual or the small group for excellence of work and hence little incentive to increase productivity. To struggle in any systematic fashion with psychosocial instrumentalities for purposes of raising or even maintaining staff motivation has been more than most general hospitals have felt they could undertake, particularly when they did not have so much as one research psychologist or other social scientist to assist them.

They have felt somewhat better prepared to work with the other factor in the above equation, namely, that of aptitude. As a result most large institutions now have personnel departments that are demonstrating progressive ability to select staff with more discrimination. Many hospitals, moreover, are in the process of enlarging their in-service training and their staff education programs under the guidance of qualified teachers, and are attempting to strengthen the amount and the competence of the supervision provided. Although these efforts are focused primarily on raising the aptitude of staff, some of them may have an indirect effect on motivation. Occasionally, at least, educational programs and supervision of a counseling nature are being consciously used in part for motivational purposes.

It is a thesis of this monograph that motivation presents a problem, particularly for large hospitals, that is often scarcely less important than that of shortages of staff. Some hospital administrators have admitted that unless staff roles could be redefined and the interest of personnel in their work improved, further increase in numbers would be almost as ineffective as pouring water into a sieve. If this assumption be sound, it would seem imperative that hospitals direct more attention to methods of possible amelioration. So much of a broadly general or highly specialized nature has been written about motivation, however, and so conflicting have been many of the points of view expressed that it is not easy to find suggestions in the literature that could hopefully be applied to hospital situations without considerable testing.

Perhaps, however, we might begin with the observation that, although motivation may be uniformly high or low in a particular organization, it is likely to differ among the various groups of personnel. This appears to be true of hospitals. Hence, instead of referring to motivation as if it were an overall problem, determination of where it is strongest, where weakest, and the reasons for these differences becomes a logical first step. The next section looks at three fairly distinctive groups of staff that participate in direct patient care, and seeks to predict what level of motivation they are likely to bring to their work in the hospital and what effect the formal organization may have on it. Many of the ideas presented in this section have been taken from an article by Dr. Oswald Hall, professor of sociology at the University of Toronto, whose analysis of the reasons for difference seems highly plausible and potentially helpful.[1]

[1] "Motivation and Morale," *Hospital Administration*, vol. 4, Summer, 1959, pp. 6–20.

EFFECTS OF DIFFERENT WORK MODELS ON MOTIVATION

The first of the three groups to be described is composed of persons who have had extended academic education and professional training; the second, of those who have had varying degrees of predominantly technical training; and the third, of those engaged without any formal preparation, who may or may not be inducted into their work in the hospital through an organized program of in-service training. These groups are likely to bring quite different expectations about their role and how they will perform it, which have been largely determined by earlier work images or models. These expectations rest upon what a group has learned during training (or previous work experience) was an appropriate role, what professional or membership associations define as appropriate, and what colleagues or fellow workers imply is desirable. If their expectations are congruent with what the institution defines as the role of a particular group, motivation is likely to be good. If there is sharp lack of congruence, productivity may be low.

The Medical Profession

We shall look first at physicians, the oldest of all the health professions. They are viewed by other professions as having exceptionally high motivation. They are accustomed to work long hours often in tension-charged situations, and to have numerous and diversified interests. Yet they seem to experience less fatigue than many other persons. Both doctors and the laity have raised the interesting question of whether those who choose medicine as a career do not tend to have a physiologically higher level of energy. The social scientists would be inclined to find another explanation for their ability to sustain effort and attention: they are largely absorbed in interest in what they are doing, their work generally provides appreciable variety, and much of it involves challenging solution of problems. They have been conditioned, moreover, from the time they entered medical school to expect a very active but rewarding professional life.

The work model on which medical behavior is patterned is extensive in time and clear in outline. Physicians can turn with pride to the classical figures of Aesculapius and Hippocrates; to the ancient medical schools of Salerno, Bologna, and Paris; to the great achievements of those nineteenth century doctors who introduced modern medicine; and to the remarkable scientific and clinical advances of their own colleagues. Thus they belong to a tradition that is highly sustaining, and that is continually being reinforced by the programs of the professional associations and articles in countless journals. This tradition has incontrovertibly demonstrated its social usefulness, and has succeeded in providing its practitioners with generous financial rewards as well as broad recognition. With such a model before them physicians learn to see themselves and to expect to be seen by others as indispensable. Is it any wonder that they bring high motivation to their work in the hospital as well as elsewhere?

Except for the medical house staff, they have been able to keep themselves outside the formal organization of most general hospitals. Thus they have maintained much independence of judgment and action. As we have noted earlier, however, they are often exigent in their demands upon the hospital. Frustrating as are such experiences both for them and for the institution, their great prestige puts them generally in an advantageous position and the "rightness" of their tradition also helps to sustain them in the face of frustration.

The Newer Health Professions

The newer professions that are found within the hospital— nurses, social workers, hospital administrators, dietitians, dentists, pharmacists, physical and occupational therapists, the top echelons of laboratory staff, and sometimes social scientists—are building work models that do not differ appreciably from those of physicians. In varying degrees their models have been patterned on those of the medical profession. Their traditions are relatively much shorter, their distinguished forebears fewer, and their current achievements and status less conspicuous. But they are moving forward very much in line with professional development as it has evolved in this country, and their training schools are concentrating increased attention upon building systematic bodies of knowledge and methods of research that can be taught to future practitioners. Their formal training, membership in professional associations, and contacts with colleagues all tend to reinforce the image of themselves as self-motivating, if not self-controlling; socially useful and often indispensable; desirous of opportunity for continued development; and eager for recognition of the importance of their contribution from the other professions with which they work.

Unlike physicians, few of the members of these groups are associated with hospitals as independent practitioners. Aside from private duty nurses who are declining in numbers, and some dentists and pharmacists, almost everyone is employed on a salary basis and comes within the formal organization and social system of the institution.

It has generally been assumed—perhaps because of the long dominance of the medical and legal professions and of the clergy —that one of the characteristics of professions is the desire of their members to be self-controlling.[1] To the extent that that assumption is true, such persons can scarcely like to fill organizational "line" positions within the chain of command where they must assume duties and responsibilities necessary to maintain the institution. Such positions may be particularly distasteful to them if the top administrative posts are occupied by men or women representing fields of competence other than their own. This fact might well tend to dampen motivation, were it not possible for most of these groups to view themselves as independent in considerable degree of the authority of the hospital. Those who work with patients on an individual basis or in special areas of the hospital separate from the patient floors, may see themselves primarily as *therapists* whose chief identification is with "their" patients or with the referring physician rather than with the institution. Although the problem of hospital control is thus minimized, they still have the fact to face of working under medical orders, which again reduces their exercise of self-control. Some of these professions appear to chafe more under such restrictions than do others.

[1] Solomon, David N., "Professional Persons in Bureaucratic Organizations" in *Symposium on Preventive and Social Psychiatry*, April 15–17, 1957, Walter Reed Army Institute of Research. Government Printing Office, Washington, pp. 253–264.

One factor must be taken into consideration, to which the literature of the professions has as yet perhaps given inadequate attention. The concepts of independent practice and professional self-control are undergoing great change as new work models, more in conformity with the growth of large institutions, are appearing. Professional persons, including even physicians and lawyers, are progressively entering large bureaucratic organizations where more of them now occupy line positions than formerly. The training for the newer professions reflects this trend. Students are increasingly conditioned from the beginning to see themselves and their future work as an essential but integral part of organized efforts to provide service through the pooling of many kinds of human and material resources. Thus they come to the hospital with some degree of expectation of being within its social system. Their motivation is likely to depend not so much on determining *what* they will do as on being self-directing in *how* they will do the tasks within their area of responsibility and on having leeway to expand that area. They want to gain satisfaction and recognition, including advancement, from working close to the highest level of their competence; they believe that the other professions and hospital administration know too little about the scope of their training and experience to pass effective judgment on what the boundaries of their areas of responsibility should be.

A special word must be said about the nursing profession since it, par excellence, has long occupied line positions stemming directly from the hospital administration. Aside from private-duty nurses, clinical instructors, and an occasional nursing consultant, the nursing service of a hospital has had few opportunities to view itself as independent in any considerable measure of institutional controls. Because nurses on all the administrative and supervisory levels are charged with much of the responsibility for running the patient areas, they must identify themselves with the goals of the institution and attempt to promote its interests, as well as those of the patients. When one recalls, in addition, that nurses also work under medical direction, and have rarely been given authority commensurate with their responsibility, one can only conclude that they have assumed their duties with remarkable equanimity. They have performed them with great loyalty and general efficiency, if not with as much flexibility and imagination or firmness in supporting the interest of patients as have usually been needed.

Their ready willingness to occupy line positions, sharply defined by "the system," may result in part from their personality pattern to which reference was made in the preceding chapters. But in no inconsiderable part it results from the fact that all nurses until recently received their basic training in hospital schools. The educational model of such schools has been one of conditioning students to work within and to identify themselves with the institution, rather than to identify themselves with the several groups of "therapists." Even though they appear able to function under the multiple subordination characteristic of the hospital with perhaps less strain than might be expected, the high turnover of staff nurses and the frequent dissatisfaction of supervisors with the lack of significant meaning in their work point to stresses that merit attention.[1]

As more nurses receive professional training within the university, which places far greater emphasis upon autonomy for the individual than does the hospital school, will they progressively seek to free themselves from being incumbents of positions over which they exercise limited control? Already some hospitals are complaining, although generally without substantial evidence, that college graduates are taking positions in public health and community nursing agencies rather than in institutions. Some are using this "fact" as an argument for perpetuating hospital schools. If statistical data bear out their assumption, careful examination will be indicated of whether changes can be made in the hospital social system that would increase the attractiveness of nursing positions for women whose basic professional education has been in universities.

Technicians

We turn now to the second group of staff participating in direct patient care, who have received at least some formal preparation for their work.

[1] See Isabel Menzies' conclusion, reproduced as Appendix 6, about the situation in a group of London hospitals.

If any strict classification were attempted, an undetermined number of registered nurses would have to be included in this category. Although these nurses have been graduated from three-year schools, the hospitals that operate the particular schools have been so lenient in admission policies, the "academic" part of the curriculum has been so weak, and the apprenticeship element of training has been so large, that the graduates are technicians rather than professional persons. Such appreciable progress has been made, however, in closing poor schools, up-grading nursing education generally, and expanding the influence of the professional associations, that all registered nurses have been included here as members of a profession. It must be noted that several of the other health professions also include persons with limited preparation for their work, who have been admitted to membership in professional associations through having been given courtesy privileges, or, to use the familiar phrase, through having been "blanketed in."

Technicians, as the term is used in this context, consist primarily of trained practical nurses, or licensed vocational nurses as they are called in two states. (Some of the medical and laboratory technicians, who have brief but functionally important contacts with patients, would also fall within this category.) Although untrained practical nurses have long taken care of patients in homes, the advent of the licensed practical nurse in the hospital is a new phenomenon. When a few facilities for their training were initially established, it was assumed that their preparation would enable them to care for subacute, convalescent, and chronic patients; hence they would be particularly helpful in reducing the pronounced shortages of personnel in long-term hospitals, nursing homes, and patients' private homes. So great, however, were the personnel needs of hospitals for acute disease that almost immediately they began to be engaged by these institutions. Today they work predominantly in general rather than in long-term hospitals.

As a result of their demonstrated usefulness, a system of facilities for training practical nurses has been evolving throughout the United States for the past decade and a half. Currently almost 700 state-approved programs, graduating some 20,000 students annually, are in operation under a variety of auspices, chiefly vocational high schools and hospitals. Most of them admit women between the ages of eighteen and fifty, and many, particularly those in specialized hospitals, welcome men as well as women. The curriculum that is generally one-year in length consists of some four months of classroom and laboratory instruction, followed by eight months of supervised practice in hospitals and sometimes also in private or nursing homes.

Federal and state agencies have done much to sponsor and finance this vocational training. Particularly vigilant in its efforts as a promotional and standard-setting organization has been the National Association for Practical Nurse Education and Service. Recently the National League for Nursing has established a Department of Practical Nurse Programs. State membership associations of practical nurses have been developing rapidly; their annual meetings closely resemble those of professional associations. Thus, through the efforts of the training programs and the national and state associations, work models are in the process of being created that will do much to determine the expectations that licensed practical nurses bring to their work.

As viewed by the general hospital, they occupy a position intermediate in responsibility, status, and salary between that of registered nurses and nursing aides. They work under the supervision of a registered nurse but they have been taught to do a great many of the nursing procedures; except for caring for patients in acute stages of illness, they perform these procedures with a minimum of direction. Although the earlier strained relations between the registered and practical nurses are disappearing, the former group appear to think of practical nurses as *assisting them*. A different perception is being fostered among the practical nurses. They are encouraged to view themselves as the nurses who "nurse the sick" or who "nurse at the bedside." These statements imply that the registered nurses are progressively moving from the bedside into supervisory and administrative positions, or are so occupied with highly specialized tasks that they have little time to become acquainted with patients.

Because the advent of licensed practical nurses is still so recent, it is impossible to predict whether they will continue to maintain their present high level of motivation in general hospitals unless these institutions make more provision for advancement in further training, rank, and salary based on recognition of merit. They tend to fare better status-wise in hospitals for long-term disease and in nursing homes that are able to recruit so few registered nurses that they can become charge nurses and may perhaps occupy even the position of supervisor.

Health Workers Without Formal Preparation

The third category of health personnel giving direct patient care is composed of persons who have had no formal training for their job prior to entering the hospital. Some of them receive carefully planned, systematic in-service training under the direction of competent teachers. Classroom instruction accompanied by demonstrations is offered before these employees have any contact with patients; their work is then supervised closely until they are entirely familiar with the procedures they are expected to carry out and with hospital routines. Probably a much larger proportion still receive only a very brief and cursory introduction to their future tasks before being assigned to their work stations. They must learn on-the-job where the regular hospital staff show them what to do as time and interest permit.

So urgent is the need for workers of several kinds who are not available, in part because of the paucity of schools, that in-service training of an unexpected nature has been instituted in some places. Thus physical and occupational therapy assistants, dietetic assistants, and even social work assistants have made their appearance. A fairly high level of general education is prerequisite for admission to these types of positions, and often persons can be found who have in addition interest and incentive.

The large class of personnel in the third category, however, is composed of nursing aides, including orderlies; in the federal hospitals they are designated as nursing assistants; in most mental hospitals they are called attendants or psychiatric aides. In general hospitals, where they are used sparingly with patients who are acutely ill, their number is somewhat smaller than the combined figure for staff, private duty, and practical nurses. In long-term hospitals where they provide most of the ward patient care, they are perhaps five times as numerous as are such nurses.

Although many nursing aides are drawn to hospitals because they want to do something for the sick, probably much larger proportions are looking merely for a job, under the most pleasant conditions possible, whereby they can earn a living. The dignified hospital buildings, the prestige of these institutions, and the well-laundered uniforms must seem to provide a desirable setting for those with white-collar inclinations. Such persons come without any work model, created and fostered by a training school or membership association, that emphasizes the importance of emotional commitment to their work as a social obligation, or as a prerequisite to personal growth and development and to possible advancement on the job. Instead, they are likely to come with ready suspicion of persons in supervisory positions.

Because they are primarily interested in the pay envelope, they have little identification with the goals of the institution. Their identification (always excepting those individuals who gain real satisfaction from taking care of patients) is largely restricted to their fellow workers. Unless they are able to develop strong ties with a small work group that has some positive orientation, their motivation is likely to be low and their chief concern is in getting through the shift without "wearing themselves out."

The unfortunate results of this attitude in lack of attention to patients has been made abundantly clear in illustrations presented earlier. It should not be thought, however, that these workers consciously intend to neglect patients or to expend the least energy possible. Where motivation is low, they experience decreased perceptivity and sensitivity: they do not *see* things that need to be done; they cannot feel how distressing it is to patients in pain to have to wait for small services or to be handled with other than great gentleness. They frequently feel so "dragged out" themselves, moreover, that they readily exaggerate the amount of work they have accomplished or that is expected of them.

To complicate the picture further, large proportions of the nursing aides in many parts of the United States are drawn from minority groups that are suffering from strong feelings of insecurity, if not of hostility. They are often in acute need of massive doses of praise, reassurance, and a form of recognition that gives them the sense of being accepted as human beings without prejudice or unfavorable discrimination. Many individuals in these groups appear to supervisory staff who are without psycho-social orientation in working with them, to have a "chip on their shoulders," to be oversensitive and resentful, or to be far too deferential or "stand-offish." Hence, instead of giving them the psychological support they need, it is easy for staff and head nurses unconsciously to withdraw from them, much as is often done with "uncooperative" patients. The medical staff, it has been noted earlier, are rarely acquainted with the nursing aides, except perhaps the orderlies. The result of withdrawal and neglect only reinforces a feeling of being rejected.

Because this subject is so important in its potential implications for patient care but has received no attention earlier in the monograph, we wish to give an illustration of the problem as viewed by an educated and perceptive patient. We then wish to comment on the fact that some hospitals have gone far toward solving the problem.

On the large male neurological ward of a long-term hospital, practically all of the nursing care except for medications and a few specialized treatments or procedures was given by men aides. Over and again one of the patients analyzed for the writer why he believed the care was so meager and careless in spite of the generous number of aides employed. Never once did he question the fundamental ability of most of these Puerto Rican and Negro men or the adequacy of the in-service training that had been given them. The problem lay in the fact, he was convinced, that almost no one paid any attention to them as individuals. He insisted that, if he were physically able, he would like the opportunity of attempting to see whether he could establish a psychological climate whereby a group of such aides might turn more of their energy outward for constructive purposes, and might finally come to be willing to make an emotional commit-ment to their work.

An occasional hospital at least has succeeded in capitalizing on the community report that it provided a better work situation for mem-bers of minority groups than was available elsewhere. Some of the Veterans Administration hospitals, with their policy of nonsegrega-tion and their increasing skill in using psychological methods for gaining the interest and support of employees, have achieved a rela-tively stable, efficient, and well-motivated class of nursing assistants.[1]

[1] For further details see Esther Lucile Brown's "The Nursing Profession and Aux-iliary Personnel" in *Aspects of Public Health Nursing*, World Health Organization, Geneva, 1961, pp. 25–28.

This has frequently occurred in those very parts of the nation where the minority group or groups felt most disadvantaged. The achievement, however, is not always easy to maintain. As one psychiatrist pointed out, let the newspaper or radio report some community incident that stirs anxiety and tension within the members of the minority group, and the result may be seen quickly reflected in the tendency of the aides to withdraw from spontaneous participation in intergroup contacts in the hospital.

DIFFERENTIATED ATTEMPTS TO STIMULATE MOTIVATION

From the foregoing discussion it would appear that the question of motivation of hospital staff has two fairly distinctive facets, and hence very different ways of handling these facets may need to be found. Physicians rarely present a problem of motivation, except in hospitals where the house staff are so badly paid or so overworked that there have been recent outbursts of discontent, and in a few public hospitals where tired, run-down doctors have found a salaried haven for themselves.

For those other health occupations moving toward complete professionalization, a sense of individual and group achievement is of vital importance. Their conditioning leads them to expect considerable freedom to exercise initiative and independence of judgment in the ways whereby they carry out their designated responsibilities and in the definition of their areas of competence. As has been suggested, many of them want to be viewed as therapists (or evolving therapists) with specialized bodies of knowledge and skills, rather than simply as therapeutic or technical assistants. Hence they believe that they should be permitted both individually and collectively to share in the planning and making of decisions that involve aspects of the therapeutic process.

In the instance of nurses, they are generally willing to act as assistants to physicians and to hospital administrators provided they be given some latitude and recognition in so acting, and *provided the central core of nursing be viewed as a unique contribution to patient care and the protection of health that is neither an extension of medical practice nor of hospital administration.*[1]

---

[1] Johnson, Dorothy E., "The Significance of Nursing Care," *American Journal of Nursing*, vol. 61, November, 1961, pp. 63–66.

It is our assumption that for all of these groups, as for professions generally, the most profound motivation to work comes from a sense of accomplishment in the position held, a feeling of personal growth through assuming responsibility that is matched by an appropriate degree of authority, and opportunity for advancement. These groups are composed of individuals, large numbers of whom seek self-actualization or self-realization through their work. It is only through the performance of tasks that they can accomplish something that fulfills their aspirations for achievement; it is only through accomplishment that they can hope for professional approval or recognition from their colleagues and the hospital. As the process of professionalization develops further and work models become stronger and more incisive, the desire for self-actualization through work that can be categorized as truly professional is likely to increase in strength and to encompass still larger proportions of these groups.

If such assumptions have validity, institutions concerned with maintaining or raising the level of motivation of their professional personnel should probably give major attention to whether the work is or *can* be made interesting and challenging for the various groups involved, and whether adequate opportunities for advancement exist or *can* be created. All other efforts are probably of secondary importance for this category of staff, except one that is necessitated by the special nature of the hospital. We refer to the need described in the first chapter for providing psychological support to those persons who find themselves in situations likely to create considerable anxiety. We shall return to this subject later.

Some support of a research nature for the assumption that what professional persons want most from their work is a sense of self-actualization, comes from the excellent small book, *The Motivation to Work*, prepared by Frederick Herzberg, Bernard Mausner, and Barbara Bloch Snyderman, and published in 1959. Unfortunately, we do not know what the possible degree of applicability of their study of some 200 engineers and accountants, associated with industrial concerns that produced and fabricated metals, may be to professional groups in hospitals. Their data and interpretations are so rich, however, if only for suggestive purposes, that a digest is being presented here.

Each of the engineers and accountants interviewed was asked to recall at least one time when he felt "exceptionally good" and one when he felt "exceptionally bad" about his job. In addition to the descriptions thus obtained, the interviewers probed their respondents about attitudinal effects on a deeper level. When the results of the data were analyzed, *achievement* stood in first place in the reports of positive job-attitudes. No fewer than 41 per cent of the respondents had told stories that emphasized successful completion of a piece of work. Recognition stood in second place; 33 per cent mentioned it. Work itself was in third place followed by responsibility, and then advancement. Salary gained sixth place, with 15 per cent mentioning it. Then followed ten factors, including interpersonal relations, that appeared at most in 6 per cent of the reports.

The authors' summary of their "several clear-cut findings" from the descriptions of positive job attitudes reads in part as follows: "First, only a small number of factors, and these highly interrelated, are responsible for good feelings about the job. Second, all of the factors responsible for good feelings about the job relate to the doing of the job itself or to the intrinsic content of the job rather than to the context in which the job is done. Third, the good feelings about the job stemming from these factors are predominantly lasting rather than temporary in nature. Fourth, when good feelings about the job are temporary in nature, they stem from specific achievements and recognition of these specific achievements. Fifth, an analysis of second-level factors [reasons given by the respondents for their feelings] leads us to the conclusion that a sense of personal growth and of self-actualization is the key to an understanding of positive feelings about the job. We would define the first-level factors [description of objective occurrences] of achievement, responsibility, work itself, and advancement as a complex of factors leading to this sense of personal growth and self-actualization. In a later discussion of these data we postulate a basic need for these goals as a central phenomenon in understanding job attitudes."[1]

When an analysis was made of the descriptions of periods during which these engineers and accountants had felt "exceptionally bad" about their job, the factors determining their feelings proved to be very different. Company policy and administration was the single most important factor; one-third of the respondents mentioned it. Two aspects of this factor were apparent. In the first kind of story, inefficiency, waste, duplication of effort, and a struggle for power were emphasized; in the second, emphasis was placed not so much on the ineffectiveness of the company as on the deleterious

---

[1] Herzberg, Mausner, and Snyderman, *The Motivation to Work.* John Wiley and Sons, New York, 1959, p. 70.

effects of its policies. These included personnel and salary policies that were frequently seen as unfair. Supervision was second among the factors. Throughout the many criticisms of it, the supervisor's lack of competence in carrying out his function appeared in 20 per cent of the descriptions; poor interpersonal relations with supervisors appeared in 15 per cent. Work itself was a factor in negative attitudes in 14 per cent of the stories: the work was routine and did not permit a man to use his creative abilities, or opportunities to learn and expand his scope were minimal. More workers complained of too little work than too much. Working conditions came in for some criticism, as did failure to get an anticipated promotion.

A study of the data contrasting factors that caused negative attitudes with those that produced positive ones leads to some interesting and perhaps very significant conclusions. Herzberg, Mausner, and Snyderman believe their evidence demonstrates that a great many things can be the source of dissatisfaction, whereas the factors that produce positive job attitudes are almost exclusively limited to achievement, recognition, work itself, responsibility, and advancement. Moreover, achievement and recognition, the two most frequently occurring factors, they see as of short-range value in creating satisfaction, while work itself, responsibility, and advancement stand out as the long-range sources of satisfaction.

The reports of negative job attitudes contained references to these five factors to be sure, although in much smaller percentages than in the stories of positive attitudes. Interestingly, achievement and responsibility appeared in only 7 and 6 per cent respectively; apparently the role of these factors in producing low job satisfaction is very small. Company policy and administration, supervision, and working conditions, which are the major sources of dissatisfaction, have little potency to affect job attitudes in a positive direction. Salary, the one item that appeared with equal frequency in both types of descriptions, seems to have more potency to cause dissatisfaction than satisfaction.

To summarize their conclusions, the authors write: "Job satisfiers deal with the factors involved in doing the job, whereas the job dissatisfiers deal with the factors that define the job content. Poor working conditions, bad company policies and administration, and bad supervision will lead to job dissatisfaction. Good company policies, good administration, good supervision, and good working conditions will not lead to positive job attitudes. In opposition to this . . . recognition, achievement, interesting work, responsibility, and advancement all lead to positive job attitudes. Their absence will much less frequently lead to job dissatisfaction."[1]

[1] *Ibid.*, p. 82.

Stimulating Motivation Among the Auxiliary Personnel

Having attempted to examine what might best stimulate motivation among the professional groups, we must now turn to the auxiliary personnel who constitute the second facet of the problem. Most of these persons probably do not expect to find satisfaction in their work. This fact, coupled with their frequent hostility toward but dependence upon those who exercise authority, often makes stimulation exceedingly difficult. They see themselves as having to be deferential to all staff in superior positions when no one is deferential to them; in general, they are keenly aware of the fact that they represent the lowest rung of the ladder in prestige, opportunity for advancement, or even consideration shown them. Hence job dissatisfaction tends to be frequent. It is expressed as complaints against their supervisors, pay, working conditions, amount of work expected of them, or by unnecessary absenteeism and rapid turnover. Dissatisfaction revolves around those factors described in the preceding section that define the job context.

It is for just such persons as nursing aides whose jobs are usually atomized, cut and dried, and monotonous that careful attention needs to be paid to what Herzberg, Mausner, and Snyderman call the factors of "hygiene." Hygiene, these writers point out, is not curative but rather preventive. "Similarly when there are deleterious factors in the context of the job, they serve to bring about poor job attitudes. Improvements in these factors of hygiene will serve to remove the impediments to positive job attitudes."[1] Among the factors enumerated are supervision, interpersonal relations, physical working conditions, administrative practices, compensation including benefits, and job security.

The purpose of concentrated attention to these factors, as viewed by these authors as well as other social scientists interested in industrial relations, is to make work "tolerable" for those persons whose jobs are fundamentally monotonous and uninteresting. We would agree that success in making work tolerable would in itself be a considerable accomplishment. Before closing this

[1] *Ibid.*, p. 113.

discussion, however, we wish to ask very directly the question that has been implied several times in this monograph. Is it not possible to make work a little more than tolerable for considerable segments of auxiliary personnel, even though they come to their jobs without any model of emotional commitment or without the motivation of those individual persons who feel a need to care for the sick? If this question can be answered in the affirmative, it changes the complexion of the problem appreciably. It not only brightens the picture for the workers, but quite as importantly it offers some promise of larger attention to, and better interpersonal relations with, patients by the group most frequently in contact with them.

Systematic experiments in improving motivation among nursing aides in general hospitals, accompanied by evaluations of the results achieved, are greatly needed. Short of such studies, a few hypotheses and enough empirical data are available to suggest a moderate degree of optimism. The stable and cohesive small work group, supported and guided by the hospital, has been referred to as one potentiality. Efforts to convince nursing assistants of their importance in patient rehabilitation illustrated an empirical undertaking. The success of some of the Veterans Administration hospitals in developing efficient and well-motivated aides, in spite of the fact that many of the latter were handicapped by membership in minority groups, has also been cited.

Psychiatrists and clinical psychologists have now had considerable experience, chiefly in psychiatric hospitals, in working with small groups of staff through informal discussion, sometimes including role-playing or psychodrama.[1] As a result of their experience they would probably agree that lack of interest or negative attitudes can frequently be reversed to the great benefit both of aides and patients. The training of supervisors in "human relations," as well as better preparation in the customary aspects of supervision, offers another possibility. Some members of the

[1] As illustration, see *Experiencing the Patient's Day* prepared by Dr. Robert H. Hyde, in collaboration with the Attendants of Boston Psychopathic Hospital, G. P. Putnam's Sons, New York, 1955.

nursing profession are now beginning to be offered such training. The applicability of skills as taught in courses on human relations to the problem of poorly motivated personnel warrants immediate and careful examination.

There are other possibilities, which do not rest so largely upon the application of knowledge from the behavioral sciences, that seem to have been little cultivated by hospitals. Engineers, who have attended special short courses in how to use competition for increasing productivity, express surprise that hospitals have not utilized this instrumentality more extensively. Competition between two or more small work groups, wards, or floors around designated tasks can frequently create marked stimulation for at least a limited period.[1] The factors in the competition must, however, be changed at fairly frequent intervals. "Projects" to be completed in specified lengths of time will frequently rally the enthusiasm of the entire staff of a unit, particularly if the projects have been given publicity throughout the hospital. Even ward bulletin boards where simple graphs and figures record accomplished tasks, as well as items in the hospital news sheet, can be used to foster interest. Certainly a wide variety of methods could be found for the purpose of relieving auxiliary personnel from some of the monotony of their work and of offering them visible evidence that what they have accomplished is recognized by others.

Giving them some voice in the planning of competitive undertakings and projects, as well as in decision-making about the ongoing work of the ward, might well be the most important source of incentive.[2] General hospitals have often been negligent in realizing that nursing aides are convinced that they frequently know more about ward conditions and certain patients than does the head nurse, or that they have sources of information at their disposal that she does not have. They want to be consulted, to have their opinion asked, to have some opportunity to express their ideas when decisions are being made that will affect them.

[1] Greenblatt, Milton, Richard H. York, and Esther Lucile Brown, *From Custodial to Therapeutic Patient Care in Mental Hospitals.* Russell Sage Foundation, New York, 1955, p. 336.

[2] Von Mering, Otto, and Stanley H. King, *Remotivating the Mental Patient.* Russell Sage Foundation, New York, 1957, pp. 184–193.

Where "team nursing" including frequent conferences about each patient has been fully and successfully introduced,[1] aides as well as practical nurses have an excellent opportunity to present their observations and offer suggestions. But these conferences are not designed for making decisions about many matters of concern to auxiliary personnel. To help them achieve enough freedom to speak in meetings where "status" persons are present, even in those places that encourage aides to attend, can be a slow and painful process. Many group leaders with experience believe, however, that if such participation is achieved aides may be able to perceive themselves as other than persons on the bottom rung.

[1] Kron, Thora, *Nursing Team Leadership.* W. B. Saunders Co., Philadelphia, 1961.

Chapter 6

EFFECTING CHANGE—I

In these two final chapters an attempt will be made, in part through summarizing some of what has already been said, to present suggestions about ways in which psychological support of staff might be strengthened in the hope that greater competence, self-confidence, and incentive would be reflected in larger interest and understanding of patients. The suggestions have been drawn from the literature of the health services, reports about and observations of recent undertakings in many hospitals, social science concepts, and experimental studies and theoretical conclusions concerning industrial and business management that seem to have relevance for hospital administration.

Some of the proposals could be initiated almost immediately; in many instances efforts already under way, at least in tenuous form or in parts of hospitals, would only need to be strengthened and developed further or extended to broader areas of the institution. These proposals will be presented first. Other suggestions deal with reconsideration of current philosophies and practices. They would require much study, discussion, and long-range planning were they to be implemented. Their application to psychological support of staff may appear less direct but the indirect effect might be substantial.

As introduction to these suggestions it is essential to restate more explicitly a point of view expressed earlier. Unless it can be done convincingly, many readers might conclude that the suggested changes would so weaken the authority structure of the hospital that they cannot be taken seriously. These readers would say that because the hospital by its very nature is concerned with the lives of human beings, certain kinds of experimental undertakings and provision for more staff freedom, which would be permissible and perhaps desirable in industry and business, cannot be tolerated. We would agree. In matters of life and death strict authority is required; we believe that the necessity for such authority is also widely accepted as a principle. The problem is not with authority per se. It is with perceptions and feelings regarding what many persons interpret as authoritarianism or the drive for power rather than authority.

To the behavioral scientists some of the aspects of the hierarchical structure of the hospital appear to foster the perception, if not the reality, of authoritarianism, and actually to weaken authority.[1] For example, the proliferation of written rules and regulations prepared expressly to minimize risk may, in fact, increase risk. This form of control can readily give administration an unjustified sense of security unless it realizes that some of the staff will almost inevitably reject these regulations with their prolixity and their seeming implication that no one except management is capable of making such decisions. "Recent psychological work has confirmed the view that externally imposed discipline is clearly inferior in results to self-discipline, and that imposed discipline tends to increase the risk of mistakes, because it does not develop individual responsibility and initiative."[2]

To use another example, the practice of grouping each profession or service and its auxiliary personnel separately under a director charged with administrative responsibility, results in such problems of communication and rivalry that essential plans for patient care not infrequently fail to be coordinated at the point of action.

Authority is essential; how to achieve its actuality represents one of the severest tests with which the hospital is faced. The suggestions noted below scarcely touch the central core of this problem. They do, however, have a bearing on some of its

[1] For a provocative discussion of how a strong person in charge of the distribution of inadequate supplies and maintenance services can wield harmful power over an entire institution and break down the established pattern of authority, see "The Locus of Power in a Large Mental Hospital" by Elaine and John Cumming in *Psychiatry*, vol. 19, November, 1956, pp. 361–369.

[2] From an unpublished paper read by Dr. A. T. M. Wilson at the 1951 Summer School, Cassel Hospital for Functional Nervous Disorders, Richmond, Surrey, England.

peripheral aspects. As such they are intended certainly not to weaken but hopefully to strengthen the structure of authority. They are intended particularly to strengthen the structure of confidence which is a necessary concomitant of authority.

STAFF'S REQUEST FOR MORE "INFORMATION"

A seemingly simple request that one hears mentioned explicitly or implicitly by all categories of staff on all levels is the request for more "information." It was illustrated earlier in the complaint of head nurses that supervisors did not tell them enough about contemplated plans or decisions made for them to work most effectively. Generally the information desired is not about rules and regulations, since those can usually be found in the procedure books. Sometimes, however, staff complain that there is no established rule or procedure to follow and there is no medical or nursing supervisor at hand to consult. Some of these complaints are entirely justified; others appear to reflect the tendency to dependency and the reluctance to assume individual responsibility that any hierarchical system is likely to foster.

What staff are chiefly asking for when they say they want more information is a wider knowledge of the context in which they work and the meaning of what they are doing. Hospitals continuously add new personnel, whether as students or regularly employed staff. Orientation to the institution is rarely extensive enough to give them the diversity of information and the consequent sense of security that they need. Even within the professional groups, moreover, individuals are often on widely varying levels of development. Some want more information because their training and experience have been inadequate for what is expected of them. Others want more just because they are farther advanced and with each increment of knowledge or understanding questions arise.

Most significant of all is the fact that rapid and continuous developments are occurring in medicine and the technological aspects of patient care. With the advent of every new and complex machine or method of diagnosis and treatment, including the highly specialized forms of surgical intervention, careful demonstration and trial practice are necessary before staff can have the skill or the confidence necessary for playing their respective roles.

Is it any wonder, in the face of these and many other factors, that staff want more information? Although their requests generally are phrased as if they were asking only to know how something is done and why, they are frequently asking in addition for reassurance and psychological support. Many times, however, they may not even be aware of this fact. The relationship between knowledge and skill on the one hand and self-confidence on the other is close—closer in specific clinical situations than is always appreciated. Supervisors may hear requests that they rightly interpret as appeals for support. Perhaps they conclude that a few words of encouragement are indicated, when what the applicant needs is help with an alarming procedure that has never been sufficiently discussed with him or in which he has had sufficient practice.

We should like to give two illustrations of how interrelated are lack of knowledge or skill and personal anxiety, and the consequent inability of the staff to provide patients with greatly needed reassurance. The first was prepared for the writer some years ago by a social scientist who has been a participant observer in countless staff conferences and clinical training sessions in teaching hospitals. Although nurses in the meantime have perhaps had better preparation for their role in connection with electric shock treatment, the use of which has also decreased since the advent of the tranquillizing drugs, the generalizations would undoubtedly be applicable to other new procedures.

> Yesterday I sat in on a class in graduate psychiatric nursing, and was struck by the extent to which nurses apparently have to engage in routines which they do not understand, and of which they do not always approve. This was a discussion group, and the talk centered around the question of how a nurse can reassure a patient who is about to undergo electric shock treatment and is uneasy about it. As the discussion progressed, it gradually became apparent that every one of the nurses there was very fearful of shock treatment. One even said, "I'd rather die than take that treatment." No one could possibly reassure patients about something for which she herself felt so strong a fear.

A few questions brought out the fact that not a single nurse in the class had ever had shock treatment explained to her in detail; that many had serious doubts as to whether it really helps patients; and that nowhere in their training program was there an opportunity to question a psychiatrist freely to learn exactly what the medical profession thinks about the treatment. It set me wondering how many other techniques and procedures there may be which those using them do not understand or may be fearful about.

The second illustration is an excerpt from a penetrating article that has been recently published. It was written by a widely known professor of pediatric nursing, following a year spent in the study of nursing care of children who have had open-heart surgery.

> Prior to taking care of Suzie, I had had a succession of short clinical experiences with other children undergoing open-heart surgery—experiences in which I needed a tremendous amount of help and support from competent staff nurses and doctors before I could even begin to function as a helping person.
>
> I was frightened by the responsibility I was carrying and knew I needed help to learn the myriad details of nursing necessary to care for these children. For example, when rereading the notes I recorded before my study of Suzie, I learn infinitely more about *me* than I do about the children who had had their hearts repaired. I needed much more experience before I could be free to see the individuality of the child, before I could relate to the child more than to the equipment and routine procedures. It was not that I was oblivious to the child's need for emotional support; it was because I could not give it until I had mastered the skills necessary to provide the physically protective nursing care required.
>
> During these experiences, the awareness of my own anxiety and of the incapacitating fear of the parents, whom I could not adequately help because of my own inexperience, became acute. My awareness of the demands of the hospital culture and of the struggle acutely ill children have in coping with these demands also became intensified.[1]

Requests for information often convey additional desires besides those for more contextual facts and "know how" or for psychological support in anxiety-inducing situations. Some clearly

[1] Blake, Florence, "In Quest of Hope and Autonomy," *Nursing Forum*, vol. 1, Winter, 1961–1962, p. 10.

suggest the desire on the part of the persons making the request for recognition of themselves and the importance of their work; others indicate the desire for closer association with colleagues above them in the hierarchical scale or with representatives of other professions, particularly physicians. Still others hint that through enlarged sources of information work could be made more interesting, or productivity and a sense of accomplishment greatly increased. Finally, many seem to intimate that the individual or the work group would like not only to be informed about developments, but to be consulted and given a voice in decisions concerning matters relevant to them or "their" patients.

When one listens carefully to these unending comments, he concludes that large sectors of personnel feel free to ask only in a very indirect, although often extremely critical, manner that perfectly legitimate and perhaps crucially important needs be met. In the light of what has been said about the almost universal desire for upward communication, the significance of extending decision-making to larger numbers, and the meaning of work, accomplishment, and responsibility as sources of motivation, cues such as these are too urgent for hospitals to ignore them.

MEETING THE REQUEST FOR "INFORMATION"

It is suggested, therefore, that hospitals introduce a wider variety of carefully planned and competently administered provisions designed to meet more fully the staff's request for "information," both in the explicit and the implicit meanings of that term. These provisions would have to go well beyond the brief and highly formalized orientation, and the sparse or random forms of subsequent staff development now sponsored by large numbers of general hospitals.

Orientation and Continuing Staff Development

Below are four recommendations recently made by official bodies in New York City pertaining to the initial orientation and in-service training of all teachers connected with the public school system. The principles set down would seem equally applicable to those categories of hospital staff that work directly with patients.

> Provide teachers and supervisors with a richer program of pre-assignment orientation.
> Upgrade materials and programs now used for orientation of new teachers.
> Develop a more effective in-service training program for all school personnel.
> Organize an in-service training program for teachers that will emphasize improvement of instruction and growth in subject matter.[1]

The initial orientation, including particularly in-service training for personnel who have had no formal preparation, needs to include not only an introduction to the program and procedures of the particular hospital, but to the specific knowledge and skills required in the positions to which the individuals are to be assigned. Even highly experienced persons often have anxiety, as did Professor Blake, about procedures new to them; many of these persons, unlike her, do not feel free to admit their inadequacies. Hence provision for extensive assistance during the early weeks might pay rich dividends in the competence and comfort of new staff.[2]

This initial period can also be used for other perhaps equally important ends of a psychological nature. At this time a level of expectation will almost inevitably be set concerning how the institution is likely to perceive the new staff and how they will perceive the hospital and its patients.[3] Discussion directly and

[1] *New York Times,* January 15, 1962, p. 14.

[2] In "Content and Consequences of an Inservice Education Program" published in the January, 1962, issue of *The American Journal of Nursing,* Ruth Barney Fine and Catherine Vavra describe the orientation and developmental programs planned for the nursing staff at the new University of Washington Hospital. They recognized the opportunity provided "to incorporate the principles of team nursing in the daily care of patients and to create an exemplary inservice teaching program." The prospective staff, coming from all parts of the United States "must be molded into an effective group, of high morale, secure in their jobs, and working as a team toward the best nursing care." (p. 54) Imaginative Procedure Fairs acquainted the staff with the complicated new equipment.

[3] For an exceptionally helpful guide to designing a program of basic instruction for hospital aides, which includes suggestions of psychological methods for winning interest and developing incentive among aides, see *Program Guide: Nursing Service,* issued by the Department of Medicine and Surgery, Veterans Administration, Washington, November, 1955. See also the *Program Guide* issued in April, 1957, on Planning a Nursing Care Program. Because this *Guide* was written to help nurses plan and evaluate the care given on patient units in conformity with current ideas about an enlarged nursing role, it could be particularly helpful as a text for discussion in continuing staff education groups.

indirectly can be focused on the subject of attitudes of staff toward patients, toward each other, and toward those in supervisory positions. Discussion of the scope of tasks to be undertaken provides ample opportunity for underlining the importance of these tasks, and hence the importance of the individual, to patient welfare and team effort. Consideration of how these tasks form an integral part of larger segments of patient care permits exploration of interrelationships with other categories of staff and existing or needed channels of communication.[1]

But no matter how successful the orientation may be, dynamic developments in medicine, concepts of comprehensive patient care, and current interest in automation demand that the program of staff education be a continuous one. Time must be made available for staff to attend; once available, staff should be expected to be present at scheduled lectures and discussions, films, demonstrations, or clinical conferences, according to the applicability of the subject. Even in hospitals that have attempted to operate good staff education programs, attendance has often been most unsatisfactory because staff did not "have time," or they thought the subject of no particular concern of theirs, or they felt that they were being invited from courtesy only. Greater numbers of hospitals have almost no such continuing program for staff except that planned and conducted by physicians primarily for themselves.

No category or level of personnel should be left without a program in which it can participate readily or feel is its own. With the great wealth of audio-visual facilities now to be had, programs can often be made more interesting and helpful than was formerly possible, particularly for those persons with limited education. The appearance of carefully prepared films dealing with the psychological aspects of patient care has been particularly encouraging.

---

[1] In a private communication to the writer, Marjorie M. Howard has commented: "I believe staff development is a prerequisite to improved patient care. However, the glaring need in nursing as I view it today is to embrace in-service education as a way of life rather than a 'thing' which, when superimposed on an existing situation, is expected to work wonders. Assisting nurses toward internalization of this concept is the challenge which those of us in educational roles have not always successfully met. It must be met before the following can be accomplished: viewing every worker as a person, making maximum use of each worker's potential, providing instruction that is patient-centered rather than procedure-centered."

For auxiliary personnel we believe that short-term training on several progressively higher levels can be used to increase competence, tenure, and incentive. Superior performance on the job, and a request for the privilege by the individual or by the small work group in behalf of one of its members, might well be prerequisites to admission to more advanced training. Thus the opportunity for further preparation could be viewed as a form of reward. Its successful completion should probably be rewarded further, as openings occur, by advancement in status classification, salary, and responsibility.

Ward Staff Meetings

One of the potentially most important instrumentalities for providing staff on a continuous basis with the contextual information and attitudes essential for helping them with their work, enlarging horizons about their role, and coordinating their efforts at the point of action, is the ward staff meeting. In the hands of an experienced leader, it can go well beyond these goals. It becomes the place where a tightly knit work group or therapeutic team can evolve, where worries and tensions can be brought up for discussion, and where reassurance and recognition of accomplishment can be given.

The following illustration testifies to what the ward staff meeting can achieve and to the diversity of ends it can serve. In the text from which this citation is taken, Dr. Richard H. York, a clinical psychologist, is evaluating the success of a research project designed to improve the care of psychotic patients in a large mental hospital. On the ward for seriously disturbed patients, where care was provided exclusively by aides under the direction of a head nurse and a psychiatrist, seclusion of supposedly unmanageable patients had been extensively used.

> The weekly ward staff meeting was the essential means whereby seclusion could be ended and other large ward changes instituted. Through it aides were given and gave each other substantial amounts of group support, in addition to what they received individually from the physician and head nurse during daily work and from the active interest taken in them by members of the research project. It was the medium through which their conflicting feelings were resolved; where they as well as the nurses were consulted before any

significant ward decisions were made by the physician, and where each step in the evolving program was carefully considered. The fact of being systematically consulted in all matters affecting their work raised their self-esteem from its former low level, and assured the involvement and commitment that were requisite to any fair trial of the program. They began gradually to perceive their status as members of a competent, progressive ward team and to find this status more rewarding and rewarded than their former role of performing restricted, routine functions.

The importance and effect of these ward meetings can scarcely be overemphasized. Among the staff itself there was agreement that the program could not have developed so successfully, if at all, without them. One aide commented about the ward sessions, "The doctor explained the changes he had planned to us. We felt that he believed it was worth a try. Actually, the meetings give you a pretty good feeling. You can get things off your chest and the group will listen to your ideas."[1]

Because meetings of this kind have been so successfully cultivated by psychiatrists, clinical psychologists, and social workers or nurses in psychiatric hospitals, social casework agencies, and an occasional pediatric or other service, it is surprising that they have not had a wider extension to hospitals for acute disease generally. Team nursing conferences contain in embryonic form many of the elements of ward staff meetings, although the goals are more limited and the group is restricted to members of the nursing service.[2] Ideally such meetings need to be held regularly and not less frequently than once a week; they should include the total nursing staff of the unit, the physician with medical responsibility for the patients, sometimes an assistant hospital administrator, and other persons such as social workers or physical therapists who either come to the floor frequently or work with considerable numbers of the patients elsewhere.

One of the most serious problems encountered is how to schedule meetings at the least busy time of day so that the maximum number can attend, and how to make them available to the members of more than a single shift. In some hospitals an

---

[1] Greenblatt, Milton, Richard H. York, and Esther Lucile Brown, *From Custodial to Therapeutic Patient Care in Mental Hospitals*. Russell Sage Foundation, New York, 1955, pp. 301–302.

[2] Brooks, Ethel A., "Team Nursing 1961," *American Journal of Nursing*, vol. 61, April, 1961, pp. 87–92.

hour has been set aside once a week in the afternoon before the morning shift leaves and the evening shift goes on duty. In occasional instances, at least, a night supervisor has attended these meetings for the express purpose of reporting later to the night shift what was discussed and what plans were made or decisions reached, and for eliciting their comments and suggestions.

The role of nursing supervision is undergoing sharp reexamination at present in university graduate courses. Possibly future nurse supervisors who have had training in group work will conclude that they should assume responsibility for planning and perhaps leading staff meetings when and as indicated, and for acting as communication agents between shifts or groups. However that may be, the immediate question of leadership presents itself. Among each of the professions represented in the hospital, some persons certainly have the requisite personality traits and considerable experience in conducting meetings of the less formalized variety. They would find little difficulty in promoting at least some of the goals indicated. Consultation provided by thoroughly experienced group leaders would probably help them in pursuing the more psychologically oriented goals; so would short courses in group leadership now available in various places or that could be sponsored for selected persons by the hospital.[1]

One of the difficulties frequently encountered in these meetings, as we have seen earlier, is the old problem of perceptions regarding authority; persons in the lower echelons generally do not feel free to speak in the presence of persons occupying positions of direct control over them. For this reason it is sometimes not advisable for the physician or head nurse to be a group leader on home territory unless he is reasonably confident that he can work through this problem. He may, however, be able to render valuable service on another ward or in other types of meetings where he is seen not as "the boss" but as an interested person.

---

[1] Many persons have expressed great interest in the teaching methods used in training courses for leaders that are often designated as "human relations laboratories." Because there has been little except highly theoretical literature on the subject, Spencer Klaw's "Two Weeks in a T-Group," published by *Fortune* in August, 1961, is helpful. He describes in detail what occurred in the small group where he was an observer. This particular course was conducted by the National Training Laboratories, a branch of the National Education Association, for business executives.

So potentially important does the ward meeting appear as one of the major forms of continuing staff education that includes an element of psychological support, that we suggest exploration of its usefulness to a variety of particular situations. For those who have never had an opportunity to see such meetings in operation, observation would constitute a first step in the exploration. Consequently inquiry would need to be made about places where these meetings have had a considerable development in the hands of experienced persons.

Emphasis has been placed upon staff meetings associated with the patient unit because this is where the greatest number of personnel giving direct care are concentrated, and where their relationships with patients and with each other tend to extend over considerable periods of time. But the concept of the group meeting that is designed to accomplish several ends simultaneously has general application. It may be just as helpful to departments of physical therapy, social work, or dietetics that are large enough to preclude easy face-to-face contacts. It has even had gratifying results when used with specialized maintenance personnel, such as electricians and plumbers, who had seen themselves as essential to the hospital rather than to patients. Their prompt attention to ward deficits has increased when they discovered in meetings held expressly for them that they had a direct effect upon patient welfare, and that that fact was recognized by a member of the therapeutic staff.

Group Psychotherapy Sessions

Some brief reference must be made to another kind of group meeting that is perhaps capable of giving greater support to persons working in acutely anxiety-inducing situations than is the ward staff meeting. Its primary purpose is to help the participants gain some understanding of themselves and their emotional reactions, as well as understanding of those with whom they are in contact, in order that they may be better able to help patients.[1] Thus its scope is narrower than that of the ward staff

[1] For a description of how this method was used with a small group of public school administrators or consultants, see the article by the psychiatrist who was the leader, the late Dr. Leo Berman, "Mental Hygiene for Educators: Report on an Experiment Using a Combined Seminar and Group Psychotherapy Approach" in *The Psychoanalytic Review*, vol. 40, October, 1953, pp. 319–332.

meeting; its depth is correspondingly greater. Although many names are given to such sessions and the term "group psychotherapy" is often avoided because of the association of "therapy" with sick persons, the meetings are seen by psychiatrists and psychologists who have developed them as combining discussion with elements of group psychotherapy.

At these sessions no agenda are followed. The perhaps six or eight persons present are encouraged to bring up for discussion whatever problems are of most concern to them. Doubts, fears, intolerance toward certain patients, or hostility toward staff and administration may be aired without fear of reprisals. Thus destructive emotions may be kept from being repressed where they fester below consciousness, and the individual often gains some insight into why he reacts as he does to certain circumstances. Group consideration of ways for caring for particularly difficult patients, or for appraising the assets as well as the liabilities in specific situations is often able to raise the level of tolerance. Leaders of such groups report instances where sufficient "allowance" was developed for patients who had been psychologically rejected and hence badly neglected, to permit staff to give them considerate and even warm, interested care.

For staff who must care for patients with incurable cancer or other diseases in the terminal stage, for those who take care of psychotic patients or the aged where physical and mental deterioration is far advanced, and for those who find the various forms of radical surgery or other treatments very distressing to themselves—for such persons the hospital ought to make every provision possible to help them in these trying circumstances. To provide this help on a group basis, the services of a psychiatrist or other psychiatrically trained practitioner or of a thoroughly experienced chaplain would probably be essential. Unless such persons can receive generous support when and as needed, how can they be expected to provide comfort either to patients or to relatives?

Staff Studies of Patient Care

Another method for meeting the need for more information, which is frequently capable of achieving several other ends simultaneously, is the patient-oriented study. Research, whether pure or applied, has such an aura of prestige attached to it within the teaching hospitals that almost all of the professional groups now want to engage in it. Generally they want, moreover, to engage in it independently or on a truly collaborative basis, and not as minor assistants to the medical profession which has given them, they believe, too little voice in the planning and too little recognition.

The ongoing work of the hospital provides little time for regular staff, even when they have had the preparation requisite to undertake research—if that term be used to mean systematic investigation designed to test the scientific validity of stated hypotheses. But the hospital provides almost unparalleled opportunity for the staff on every service to make relatively simple but highly useful studies directly related to their work. Such studies often yield vitally needed facts from which conclusions about desirable action can be drawn; they can also do much to stimulate staff interest and to give the participants a sense of accomplishment of a generally new kind.

Exploration of scores of questions growing out of daily work situations merit attention. The following suggestions are intended merely to illustrate diversity of areas, dealing only with psychosocial factors, within each of which many relevant studies could be outlined. What forms of staff behavior appear satisfying to some kinds of patients but annoying to others? Why? What methods do physicians, nurses, physical therapists, social workers, and social scientists use for obtaining pertinent information from patients? What can each group learn from the methods used by the others that might be useful to it? How do nurses make an assessment of what form of health counseling a patient needs and how it can best be given? How often do they provide health counseling or attempt to see that it is provided? What rearrangements could be made in the physical facilities of particular patient floors that would provide more comfort and satisfaction to patients, to staff? How can communication be enlarged between physicians and nurses, between nurses and dietitians, nurses and physical therapists, nurses and social workers?

The list could be lengthened indefinitely, even without touching on those many aspects of clinical procedures that need examination. As visualized here, this kind of "research" by hospital staffs would be designed to find answers to questions and to solve problems pertinent to patient care. It would also be designed to give the greatest number of persons a possible opportunity to participate in what was considered a common effort, and not an undertaking only for those on the higher levels of status and professional preparation. Methods appropriate to studies of this kind would probably consist primarily of observation, listening, interviewing, and experiments or demonstrations, accompanied by simple techniques for recording and analyzing the data collected and for evaluating the results of the experiments.

Under observation, the mere counting and recording of how often something occurs or fails to occur could often provide facts of a surprisingly useful kind that the hospital may never have had. A social scientist once remarked only half jokingly that some day a hospital administrator would make his reputation by counting what "went on" or did not go on in his institution. He would, of course, have to be an exceptionally imaginative person, as well as one who spent much time walking the hospital floors, in order to be able to see what things, formerly neglected but having an important bearing on the function and operation of the hospital, needed to be counted.

Chapter 7

EFFECTING CHANGE—II

MEETING THE NEED FOR ACCOMPLISHMENT AND RECOGNITION

INTERESTING WORK, a sense of accomplishment, and recognition from colleagues and those in higher positions have been referred to as highly important factors in motivation. The question of how these prerequisites can be made available must now receive more direct attention. Before positive methods can be explored, however, roadblocks that first need to be removed in order to make the positive steps possible or effective, require examination.

Some insight into the nature of these roadblocks, as applied to nursing at least, has been provided by the writer's annual workshop on patient care attended by nurses in supervisory, administrative, and faculty positions. When she has asked the nurses to note what rewards or recognition they felt they had received during the preceding year either in their work situation or through their profession, their replies have been illuminating if only because of the general paucity of rewards enumerated. For some of the nurses the very idea of personal rewards through work, other than through the direct care of patients that was now denied them because of the positions occupied, seemed new and even surprising. For perhaps the largest number, the idea was certainly not new or unimportant, but few rewards could be recalled; these persons often appeared to be so frustrated by the nature and complexity of their positions that their perception of what constituted reward may have been badly warped.

A few could point to a considerable number and range of rewards, some of which were then recognized by others as having been granted them, too. Among those who saw rewards in their more diverse forms, the feeling of accomplishment or even the opportunity for accomplishment was noted. An occasional nurse pointed to forms of reward so subtle that only those with acute sensitivity could probably have distinguished them.

From these papers and discussions the writer gained an impression that has been strongly reinforced by her observations of general hospitals and by such literature on the subject as she has seen. It is that consciously planned efforts to provide staff with an opportunity to experience accomplishment and recognition have not been cultivated to anything like the degree that might be desirable. Or the institution has failed to tag its rewards with sufficient clarity so that they could not be overlooked or misinterpreted.

Instead, administrative practices persist that foster a feeling among large sections of staff that their ideas are unimportant and that they are likely to be by-passed when the plums are distributed. Often these feelings may be completely at variance with the intentions of the administration, but the practices encourage harmful divergencies in perception. These are the roadblocks that merit further examination before turning to positive methods for promoting accomplishment and recognition.

Administrative Ineptitudes

Persons acquainted with Professor Mason Haire's book, *Psychology in Management*, may recall his apt statement that when housebreaking a dog we put the "Law of Effect" into practice, but when we become involved in more complicated situations we lose track of it. The principle of learning to which he refers means that "behavior that seems not to lead to reward or seems to lead to punishment tends not to be repeated."[1] As a consequence of losing track of this principle, roadblocks to motivation are set up. Two of his illustrations, which are being reproduced here, are as applicable to hospital administration as to industrial management.

> It is not at all uncommon to hear members of management describe a situation in which two applicants for a promotion are nearly equal in merit. The poorer one, however, let us say has considerably more seniority. Although there is leeway in the contract for a promo-

[1] McGraw-Hill Book Co., New York, 1956, p. 14.

tion on the basis of merit, the man with the greater seniority is promoted, in order to avoid argument. It is not at all uncommon to hear the same people say at another time, "Our biggest problem is that people don't try hard any more, the way they used to. They used to figure that if they worked hard they'd get ahead, but now they just figure that if they wait long enough they'll be promoted, so they sweat it out rather than trying to do a good job." The members of management, in these cases, are not entitled to express surprise or dissatisfaction at their subordinates' performance. The reason the subordinates produce the kind of behavior they do is they have been trained to behave that way. They have been shown that rewards come for seniority and not for merit.[1]

*   *   *   *

When someone approaches a foreman with a suggestion about something to do, does the foreman imply by his tone and manner, "Your job is to do the work—I'll do the planning"? This can be as effective a punishment, or at least lack of reward, as many more carefully planned acts, and these small everyday occurrences are the day-by-day administrations of reward and punishment, by which the superior shapes the behavior of his subordinates. Underlying the process throughout, we have the principle of the Law of Effect.[2]

In the discussion of small work groups attention was devoted to the frequent hospital practice of shifting ward personnel from one unit to another. This is a roadblock with harmful effects for the psychological development of the small group; for those nurses and aides who do not want to move or who dislike the manner in which they are rotated, it is often viewed as a punishment.[3] How unfortunate this practice may be for the nurse who merits reward rather than punishment, and how the effect is reflected adversely in patient care, Professor Marion E. Kalkman makes very clear in the following statement.

Psychiatric nurses are taught the importance of slowly developing rapport with a patient, then using this relationship to further the patient's therapeutic progress. Yet how often has a nurse worked hard to do this with her patients only to find herself transferred to another ward. Such an action negates the value of all the work the nurse has invested in her patients. The most destructive aspect of

[1] *Ibid.*, p. 15.
[2] *Ibid.*, p. 16.
[3] See section entitled "Detachment and Denial of Feelings" in Appendix 6 of this monograph, p. 186.

such administrative action is that in the future the nurse is not likely to show as much consideration for her patients as formerly. She is too concerned with her own feelings of dissatisfaction and unhappiness to be observant of her patients' feelings and to be patient and tolerant with them. . . . Therefore, if an administrator expects her nurses to show consideration for patients, she must first demonstrate her interest in the welfare and happiness of her nurses.[1]

Distortions of Perception

Thus far the discussion has been concerned with administrative ineptitudes; these are the failures of commission as seen in the light of the psychology of management. Only somewhat less important perhaps in their effect of denying personnel a sense of accomplishment and recognition are failures of omission. Many hospitals have introduced provisions that have been designed as rewards or could justifiably be used for that end, but have failed to make that fact sufficiently explicit. Sometimes personnel have even misinterpreted the meaning of the provisions; such distortion of perception can, of course, nullify any possible effectiveness.

In the preceding chapter under the heading "Meeting the Request for Information," almost every suggestion had implicit in it a possible contribution to more than enlarging the staff's factual knowledge. Strengthening self-confidence, making provision for direct psychological support, increasing interest in the job through better preparation, greater assurance, and participation in situations such as ward staff meetings and action-oriented studies—these are some of the potentialities that could be developed and made explicit to staff. Every undertaking initiated by the hospital that permits personal growth and development of the worker can rightfully be viewed by the initiators as recognition of his worth and as a reward offered him.

Frequently administrators who have participated in such undertakings have read informative papers at professional meetings, which have created much interest and led perhaps to the conclusion that the particular hospital was in the vanguard of progressive ideas. Yet the staff of that hospital may never have

---

[1] Kalkman, Marion E., "Creative Administration" in *Examining Psychiatric Nursing Skills*. First Midwest Conference on Psychiatric Nursing, April 11–14, 1956. American Journal of Nursing Co., New York, pp. 43–48.

seen or heard of the paper, and large segments have not known that programs they took for granted were distinctive. Except for those professional persons who follow trends closely, the staff tend to conclude that the programs existing in their institution are something that all hospitals foster or ought to foster. Hence dynamic advances may fail to serve as sources of motivation for them.

Even in a small and intimate psychiatric hospital that is able to report that more than one hour of group "teaching" is provided for every hour of work with patients, it may be questioned whether the newer members of the staff know much about the years of concentrated study and effort that have gone into evolving this program. The *raison d'être* for the lavish expenditure of time and money has been stated as follows: "If one believes that high staff morale is vital, that job flexibility, autonomy, and room for creativity are important, and that patients can be reached best through well-motivated staff, these efforts appear necessary and worthwhile both to enhance the therapeutic potential of staff and to keep it at a high level."[1]

Persons reading the statement and not knowing about the generous attention that has been given in that institution to individuals as well as to staff groups, might still conclude cynically that no hospital pays for time out of consideration for personnel; its *only* interest is in making them more useful to the institution. Ways need to be found, short of the use of blatant advertising methods, for demonstrating to staff that the hospital *is* interested in them; that it realizes that only to the degree that their psychological needs are met and mutual confidence is established can it hope that they will set high goals of performance for themselves.

Many of these ways will undoubtedly have to be evolved outside the hierarchical system. It has been easy for administrators and supervisors to put plans into action that they sincerely considered for the welfare of personnel, but then forget to explain adequately the reasons for what they have done. Most often perhaps they have failed to attempt to discover before initiating

[1] Greenblatt, Milton, "Formal and Informal Groups in a Therapeutic Community." Paper read at the Annual Institute and Conference, American Group Psychotherapy Association, New York City, January 27–30, 1960.

a plan whether their perception of its desirability and outcome, and that of the staff were likely to be congruent.

Let us report the simplest kind of incident as illustration. A nursing supervisor decided that it would be good for the motivation of nursing aides if she invited several of them to accompany her to another city to hear a lecture on patient care. (Never before in that hospital had the privilege of leaving one's work to attend an out-of-town meeting been accorded to auxiliary personnel.) The supervisor asked five aides to go with her, thus filling her car to capacity. En route they stopped for lunch in a pleasant restaurant. When they reached the meeting hall, she introduced herself to the chairman and the speaker, explained that she was establishing a new precedent by bringing auxiliary rather than professional personnel to the lecture, inquired whether some announcement might be made at the meeting about the fact that the hospital had given the day off to the five aides, and said that she would like to have the speaker shake hands and chat with them during intermission. Everything proceeded according to her plan. When the announcement was made there was general applause from the audience, including the "top brass" of several hospitals who were in attendance. During intermission the speaker shook hands and gave the aides messages of greeting to convey to the other aides upon their return.

As far as the observer could tell, this occasion was highly satisfactory both for the aides and for the supervisor. It may be assumed that the latter was so experienced she had taken the steps necessary to foresee a fortunate outcome, and that she was exercising initiative and positive leadership of a high order. It is just this kind of initiative, however, that often has unfortunate consequences when a less experienced person has an excellent idea that she is able to act upon by virtue of her position, but when she fails to carry through the sequence of steps necessary to guarantee its success.

She would not only need to discuss the plan with the director of nursing service and gain the latter's consent, but with representatives of the graduate nurses as well. Otherwise they might think they were being denied a privilege that they had almost come to consider a right. Then she would be faced by the most difficult decision: should she select the aides from among those who seemed to her to merit a reward, should she ask the head nurses to select them, or should she suggest that the nursing aides on each unit choose one of their members to go as their representative? If she made the selection, could she be sure that the other aides would not look disparagingly the next morning at the supervisor's "favorites"? If she let the aide groups decide, would the head nurses feel that she had by-passed them? And would the aides interpret the permission given them to make the decision as a form of recognition of their importance to the institution?

It is questions such as these that point to the many consequential facets of even small administrative decisions. The bureaucracy of the large hospital allows the administration little choice except to act without having the needed answers to pertinent questions. But action unaccompanied by adequate consultation with staff often provokes destructive rivalry, jealousy, and acute sensitivity to possible slights; these in turn "corrode the soul." Nothing suggests more clearly the need for a less formalized social system within which exchange of opinion and of proposals can occur with some frequency and spontaneity.

DECISION-MAKING BY STAFF

This brings us to consideration of decision-making by groups of staff as a positive method for replacing an attitude of indifference or negativism with something more desirable. Improved attitudes, directed toward finding ways to solve problems and accompanied by the exercise of greater self-determination, might well produce situations through which staff could experience interesting work and a sense of achievement, and gain recognition for their accomplishments. Increasingly persons with empirical experience in working with groups of staff in hospitals, as well as students of industrial management, are coming to the conclusion that the delegation of responsibility to staff for making decisions, within certain defined areas, offers one of the most promising means for alleviating a variety of institutional ills. They hold to this conclusion although they are well aware that the initiation and maintenance of delegated decision-making also present many difficulties.

In Chapter 6 attention was given at some length to the ward staff meeting. It may be thought of as the prototype of methods for permitting and encouraging a segment of the staff to decide (within the boundaries of medical orders and hospital rulings) what should be done and how in providing patient care, and in assuming responsibility for many aspects of the physical and social environment of the institution. One of its chief virtues is the fact that it allows every person regardless of the level of his position to have his say about what he thinks is or is not appropriate. He is no longer someone who always has to take orders from superiors. These meetings also provide opportunity for a larger amount of communication focused on specific tasks or problems related to patient care. From the solution of problems can come satisfaction for staff and possible benefit for patients.

The method exemplified by the ward staff meeting can be extended to meetings on a hospital-wide basis; they can be composed of representatives ranging from two in number to delegates from all the professional and nonprofessional groups concerned with patient care.[1] The basic purpose of these meetings, within the context of our discussion, would be to find answers to questions, often through planning and engaging in experiments, that were of common concern to the departments represented. Administrators and supervisors on the highest levels of authority would certainly not be excluded; their presence as persons who were acquainted with the broader aspects of general policy and who could facilitate change through granting administrative permission, would often be desirable. These meetings, however, would be clearly designed to extend decision-making and hence responsibility to far larger numbers of personnel, most of whom were in direct contact with patients and relatives. They would be designed, in addition, to open more horizontal channels of communication in behalf of improved interpersonal relations between departments and better coordination of effort in patient care.

An earlier chapter reported on a hospital's inability to provide the early morning coffee and prune juice that a patient had requested. This was in spite of the fact that a nurse and a dietitian spent an inordinate amount of time telephoning back and forth, and probably experienced almost as much frustration as did the patient. This incident is illustrative of frequently recurring problems that seem almost to defy solution under the present system. Rarely are all the persons involved given enough facts to see the total problem; conse-

[1] For helpful suggestions about setting up and directing committees with decision-making responsibilities, see Robert F. Bales' "In Conference" in *Harvard Business Review*, vol. 32, March-April, 1954, pp. 44–50, and also "How People Interact in Conferences" in *Scientific American*, vol. 192, March, 1955, pp. 31–35.

quently they often conclude that another service or a demanding patient, neither of whom has the authority, is trying to 'order them to do something. Even when the person to whom the request is made is willing to comply he may find, as did the dietetic service, that he is blocked by failure in communication or by resentful workers within his own service.

The question now is whether a solution to such difficulties could more often be reached by the means suggested here. What is the likelihood that a small committee composed of representatives of the appropriate departments, meeting in face-to-face discussion, might learn better the nature of the problem, achieve any needed correction of their perceptions of each other, and suggest one or more possible solutions to be tried out? In this particular instance a member of hospital administration, as well as representatives of nursing and dietetics, would need to be included in the discussions. His role would be that of contributing any possible suggestions, and of giving (or seeking) approval for initiation of experiments to find if the proposals succeeded. From his participation in just such "critical incidents" he might well learn of weaknesses in the social fabric of the hospital of which he had been unaware, or which would have appeared to him in quite a different light if they had been reported by the department heads individually.

Hospitals that are not accustomed to seek solutions of problems through committees horizontally organized and composed primarily of members well below the level of directors, raise numerous and often justifiable criticisms about such a method. They comment on the excessive amount of staff time required for such an effort, and the fact that there is no time in their institution that *can* be devoted to such meetings. They are concerned about the probable disruption to established lines of authority, and to the expense that may be involved in plans that include experiments.

Such criticisms must be viewed against the existing situation. Often excessive amounts of time are now *wasted* with no positive achievement and great frustration; the damage caused to incentive from working where such conditions are frequent occurrences, and also the cost to the institution are incalculable. Quite as serious perhaps is the failure to build strong bridges linking the several departments, preferably through collaborative work on relatively simple problems, that would be ready for use in those moments of acute need experienced by all hospitals.

An assistant director of a hospital devoted much of his time for many years as leader of groups of personnel, one of which was composed of members of the total therapeutic staff. It was in this way, he frequently remarked, that the hospital came out ahead in the long run even though it took six months of weekly group discussion for the staff to talk through and finally accept some new plan. Were the same plan to be introduced suddenly by executive order, he was convinced that it would probably be so imperfectly understood and would create so much dissatisfaction, anxiety, or disorganization that its rebuilding would take more than the six months.

The Committee on Patient Care

Perhaps one of the most conclusive answers to whether a hospital can afford planning and decision-making by patient centered "task forces" that cut across departmental lines, is to be found in the report of what was achieved in one hospital. There an appointed committee was faced with the problem of demonstrating that patient care could be improved on selected wards without increased budgets or enlarged overall hospital staffs. The fact that this experiment was undertaken in a psychiatric institution does not, in our estimation, preclude its applicability to general hospitals; we have seen many large public hospitals for acute disease where such an effort might have transformed poor ward conditions within the space of a few months. Although the portion of the report presented below is detailed, a few supplementary facts and comments are needed to give the reader some knowledge of the background of the undertaking, and to help him in examining the work of the committee as a succession of steps in the *process* of effecting change.

Early in the 1950's Russell Sage Foundation decided to sponsor a two-year experiment (referred to here as the Project) that was designed to see whether ward patient care in large psychiatric hospitals could be raised through the use of social techniques to a level more nearly comparable to that provided in small teaching and research institutes. The Foundation's only financial contribution was for the salary of Dr. Richard H. York, the director, to whom reference has already been made, and for the collecting of data needed for assessment of conditions and evaluation of results.

When Dr. York began his preliminary discussions at Bedford Veterans Administration Hospital, one of the institutions selected for study, he found that the chief of staff was already attempting to increase the prestige and authority of the nursing service. Hence any experiment for improving ward patient care, concluded the chief of staff, ought to rest primarily in the hands of nurses. This conclusion was later seen to be unrealistic, inasmuch as raising the level of care even on one ward can scarcely be achieved without the assistance of many persons from other services. But it accomplished the important purpose of giving more responsibility and recognition to the service most immediately concerned. Furthermore, the steering committee that the chief of staff appointed was small and homogeneous enough to permit relative ease and dispatch in early planning. Any group of the size and diversity into which the committee gradually evolved would have had the utmost difficulty in beginning to function, even with a leader of exceptional skill.

The reader should note that the committee was also favored by having two distinct kinds of support. It had the prestige of an experimental project sponsored by a research foundation. That fact undoubtedly provided some of the initial motivation for making the nursing staff eager to demonstrate what they could do. Sponsorship was perhaps quite as important in later stages in lending additional inducement to other departments to provide assistance on the wards for patients unable to go elsewhere for occupational and recreational therapy. The second kind of support was furnished by the presence at the committee meetings both of Dr. York and of the director of educational services; the latter was there expressly as the representative of the administration to sanction, whenever possible, what proved to be large changes in roles and functions.

Without some such support it is doubtful whether any undertaking of this magnitude would have been initiated or would have had the remarkable degree of success that was achieved. But the significant conclusion is that with this assistance the committee was able to move forward with progressively less help from Dr. York, and its program had an appreciable impact on many other patient units besides those selected as experimental wards.[1] Before the end of the Project the administration of Bedford had expressed appreciative surprise, and the New England Society of Psychiatrists that toured the wards reported amazement and gratification.

The principal instrumentality that the Project created, and through which it worked increasingly and with substantial results, was the progressively enlarged steering committee. Initially this committee was composed of six persons all of whom, with one exception, represented the nursing service. The assistant chief nurse in charge of nursing education was appointed chairman, and three nursing supervisors and one supervisory aide were selected to be members. As his active representative on the committee, the chief of staff appointed the director of professional education. The contribution of the latter to the collaboration between Bedford and the Project was always important and at times decisive. In exploratory ventures of this action type, inevitable frictions develop between the sponsoring and institutional groups and between persons within those groups. With his objective knowledge of the social structure of the institution and his desire to facilitate the experiment, the director of professional education frequently assumed the role of intermediary and brought dissenting individuals together to find some solution to a particular difficulty.

Selection of wards was one of the first tasks that faced the steering committee. A few persons in the Hospital were reluctant to have experimental efforts "wasted" on chronic wards so discouraging did work with them appear. Many more, however, favored inclusion of such wards for the very reason that morale there was extremely low and also because of the preponderance of chronic cases. This problem was resolved outside the formal committee meetings, and selection was made on the basis of factual data and to include both acute and chronic wards. So radical was subsequent improvement on the latter that various members of the staff, some influential enough to further developments elsewhere, testified to a complete change in their point of view about what could be done even for severely regressed patients.

[1] Readers interested in the nature and degree of change that occurred on the wards are referred to Chapters 15 and 16 of *From Custodial to Therapeutic Patient Care in Mental Hospitals*, by Milton Greenblatt, Richard H. York, and Esther Lucile Brown, Russell Sage Foundation, New York, 1955.

No sooner had the wards been selected, however, than the committee learned that at least two psychiatrists were formulating plans of their own for ward improvement without consulting with it because they were unaware of its purpose. As a consequence, the idea was conceived of monthly task-oriented meetings to include physicians as well as ward staff. Several of the nurses were so dubious, however, about the doctors' willingness to meet with them that they did not even issue an invitation until they were later informed that these particular physicians were now sitting down with their head nurses and aides to formulate ward plans. The ward physicians were also dubious about the value of meeting with the steering committee, but when they were told that its purpose would be to discuss and assist their plans they agreed to participate. Hence, after about six weeks the steering committee was enlarged to include the two physicians from the disturbed and the "continued treatment" ward, and at least one nurse and one aide from each unit. It will be referred to hereafter as the committee for patient care. Its function was viewed as that of accomplishing change not initially through administrative techniques but through meetings devoted to group planning, stimulating action, providing mutual support, and evaluating action undertaken. Frequently the action decided upon involved administrative changes.

At the beginning the committee discussions were supposedly for the sole purpose of forwarding developments on the selected wards, and hence there seemed no reason to include personnel not directly connected with these areas or with ward administration in general. Shortly, however, it became evident that not only the rehabilitation therapists but categories of personnel seemingly far removed from direct patient care were clearly connected with what occurred on the wards. An early problem was that of persuading the rehabilitation department at once to take more patients from the wards and to send workers, such as occupational therapists, with their supplies to the wards to direct activities for patients too sick to leave. As in instances of friction between other groups that did not have a common meeting ground in the wards themselves or in the committee for patient care, ward personnel and the rehabilitation staff attributed to each other lack of interest in, and clear understanding of, the needs of patients or reluctance to cooperate whole-heartedly. Considerable rapprochement was achieved through special meetings, sponsored by the chairman of the committee and by an instructor in nursing education, at which nurses and therapists discussed their respective functions in reference to occupational and recreational activities that might be performed on the wards. Some months later the medical chief of the rehabilitation department and representatives of the sections comprising it were included in the committee to obtain their participation in the group that was striving to further ward progress.

The importance of still other hospital employees seemingly more remote from patient care also became apparent: engineers responsible for the maintenance of the wards, persons delegated to furnish the supplies, members of the record room staff who assembled and controlled use of medical histories and other data. Their importance was initially highlighted in the task-oriented meetings by the then familiar complaints from ward staffs that such employees did not understand the purposes and goals of treatment. To remedy this situation the committee formulated a tentative plan to increase their understanding, and with the support and further planning of the hospital administration a series of meetings was held designed to demonstrate how they could facilitate or hinder patient care.

During the early weeks of the original steering committee the writer [Dr. York] had assumed whatever leadership of the meetings was necessary to get the Project under way. With the first enlargement in membership he began gradually by design to relinquish this role to the committee chairman, and assumed the role of a consultant who stimulated cooperative planning and action among the various groups when needed, and who maintained a constant focus on practical problems in ward care and on the functions of each type of staff. By the end of 1952 the committee for patient care was well able to stand on its own feet. Attendance at the meetings ranged from 15 to 33 with an average of some 22 present, several of whom were interested visitors. In addition to the chairman, the administrative nurses exercised overall leadership by providing continuity as a group and by planning flexible, effective use of meetings that resulted in extending improved ward care to increasingly larger areas of the Hospital. This planning function was one that these nurses could perform extremely well, since the fact that their work cut across ward and department boundaries permitted them comparative knowledge about what needed emphasis. As far as individual meetings were concerned, the degree of participation of each group depended upon the topic and area of interest. Physicians were particularly vocal when matters of policy were being considered; aides spoke when specific ward problems were examined.

When the quantitative contribution of various groups of personnel to the discussion was analyzed for seven of the monthly meetings, it was found that that of persons representing the Project decreased from 36 per cent in 1952 to about 10 in 1953. This assumption of leadership by the hospital staff was particularly gratifying for several reasons. The Project desired to initiate only those procedures that seemed to meet the ward-care needs at Bedford and that had some chance of being institutionalized by the end of the experiment. Second, it was the writer's plan continually to anticipate early termination of any excessive dependence of the Hospital on the Project or vice versa. This seemed necessary because of the broad exploratory goals of the collaboration and the fact that the extensive alterations envisaged in ward and hospital structure would inevitably affect the patients. To withdraw provision for more satisfying ward living at the close of the experiment would do them grave injustice. Finally, since learning and practical action moved hand in hand in this exploration, major responsibility for actions taken would inevitably have to reside in the long run with the hospital staff.

Well before the end of the two-year period the question was raised of the desirability of continuing the meetings. The answer was strongly in the affirmative, and several sessions were devoted to considering what kind of constituency would best serve the entire hospital. The final decision only moved the committee for patient care still farther in the direction of becoming more inclusive. Every major department in the institution was to be represented, thus adding members from several additional groups. When the new plans were completed, the committee was composed of the chief of staff; director of professional education; chief of clinical psychology; chief of the rehabilitation department; one representative each from the medical staff, research, vocational counseling, special services, and social service; five administrative or ward head nurses each with an alternate, representing the various clinical services; and seven psychiatric aides with their alternates. The hospital director and chief of nursing service were ex-officio members. The head of nursing education was chosen chairman and the writer was asked to continue serve as a consultant. Announcement was made that all hospital personnel who wished to attend the meetings were not only invited, but would be encouraged to participate in them.

Some uncertainty was expressed when the new committee was formed about the ability of so large and disparate a group to focus attention primarily upon ward patient care. This concern has been proved unjustified. Monthly meetings are now being held at which every ward or building in the Hospital presents its program in turn. Presentations are the joint responsibility of the ward physician, head nurse, charge aide, and those special therapists working on the ward or with patients from it. The meetings have created much interest and appear to be fulfilling the major functions of the committee as now defined: to stimulate and make some assessment of patient care programs, to give support and recognition on a continuing basis to the various groups directly engaged in providing care, and to recommend specific studies or administrative changes.

Achievements of Committee

Thus far little has been said specifically about what the committee did through its meetings other than make selection of wards. Space does not permit adequate review either of the content of the sessions or the methods used to build confidence and gain consensus. A brief reference must be made to types of subjects discussed, however, if only to provide further background for an evaluation of what it accomplished. Planning for improved patient care was viewed as a joint function of the committee and the ward staffs. Consequently, attention was given to formulation of general steps to be taken, discussion of their probable effects on patient behavior, consideration of the potential contribution of other departments, and so on. The care of disturbed and of untidy patients received special thought, since both categories had been included in the experimental areas chosen. Because ward staffs were relatively large, however, the committee did not have to engage in direct decision-making for each ward as did its counterpart at Metropolitan State Hospital. Instead, the Bedford committee was in a position to focus upon broader aspects of patient care, and to contribute more than at Metropolitan to coordination of the work of the wards and other departments and to assessment of progress.

One of these broader aspects around which much discussion revolved was that of new functions and roles for ward personnel, and how such personnel could be given sufficient support to enable them to assume the larger responsibilities implicit in revised alignment of duties and status. The subject of the role of aides on the experimental wards created so much interest that the department of nursing education held special meetings with them and with nurses and aides from other parts of the Hospital in an attempt to define a generic role. Questions that were the basis for much discussion were the following: To what degree were the weekly staff meetings that had been instituted on many wards instrumental in improving interpersonal relations and clarifying goals? To what extent were everyday ward relations between nurses and aides satisfactory; to what extent were those of nurses and aides with patients therapeutic?

At intervals the committee reviewed the original statement of goals of patient care, examined what had been done thus far, and then as a group tried to make some evaluation of the results. Social science concepts were introduced in the sessions whenever they could be directly related to concrete instances. Thus, motivation, interpersonal relationships and group norms, communication, and social structure were discussed over and again. Since the sociological concept of social structure is relatively new to hospitals, continuous illustrative reference was made to the way in which that structure can handicap or facilitate patient care. To demonstrate how much is lost when it is inflexible, certain patients who were transferred frequently from ward to ward were followed through one year of hospitalization. It was found that the planning done prior to transfer and the medical records accompanying them were almost always inadequate to permit staff to provide a continuous and consistent therapeutic program. The question, for example, of how patients who became acutely disturbed were handled on wards that had formerly sent them elsewhere became in itself a topic for discussion. Finally, the implications for the rest of the Hospital of what was being learned on the experimental wards were given repeated consideration.

Obviously, the achievements of the committee for patient care extended far beyond the mere forwarding of the learning process instituted by the Project. Perhaps they can be summarized under five points: (1) Through the director of professional education as the representative of the chief of staff, the committee brought the sanction of management to pronounced changes in the functions and status of ward personnel and in procedures connected with patient care. (2) It provided a collective instrumentality for assessing ward conditions and the results of the changes instituted. Never before had there been a group closely associated with patients who had been given opportunity to express such experienced judgments and as a result to build their consensus into continuing ward patterns of action. (3) The Committee stimulated interest in improving patient care among departments and services some of which were far removed from the ward. It coordinated the work of other departments and evaluated the appropriateness of their programs not only in reference to the experiment, but increasingly to the overall needs and goals of the Hospital. (4) It brought diverse groups of personnel into closer working relationships. Persons who would not otherwise have discussed with each other the practical significance of their professions, conferred freely. This fostered communication both vertically and horizontally in Bedford's social organization. Common goals were clarified, thus helping to integrate the interests and abilities of the several groups included in the committee. (5) As progress could be reported concerning the experiment, group solidarity and individual incentive were both increased—and with these gains all types of personnel were able to assume more responsibility for patient progress. Finally, responsibility and reward were shared on a broad basis as recognition grew that staff-staff and staff-patient relationships were interconnected in positive as well as negative patterns of hospital communal life.[1]

[1] York, Richard H., "Experiments in Ward Patient Care at Bedford Veterans Administration Hospital" in Greenblatt, York, and Brown, *From Custodial to Therapeutic Patient Care in Mental Hospitals*, pp. 286–294.

PLANNING FOR THE FUTURE

Any hospital that permits a comparable degree of authority to a broad cross-section of staff for initiating and developing plans, instituting experiments, and engaging in decision-making generally, has already moved far toward modification of its social system. Even if its organization chart is still readily available, new forms of social behavior tend to reinforce the importance of horizontal as well as vertical interaction, and of assumption of more responsibility by persons below the higher levels of administration and supervision.

Actual experimentation with varied forms of organization has progressed less far in general than in psychiatric hospitals, although departments of physical medicine and rehabilitation are showing interest in such efforts. But changes in attitudes are appearing with increasing frequency. Schools of hospital administration are beginning to point to the significance of the informal social system, while the following paragraph written by the administrator of a university hospital perhaps reflects the outline of progressive thinking in such institutions.

> Emerging management concepts suggest that organizational structure should initiate from and around the job to be done, not from the top down. In the hospital, this would mean that hospital organization should be built on patient care; this implies a multidiscipline type of structure rather than departments as they exist today. Another concept that we can well ponder is one that suggests the organizational structure should contain the least possible number of management levels with the shortest possible chain of command.[1]

One of the great tasks immediately ahead is that of attempting to see how means can be evolved, to fit the requirements of different kinds of hospitals, that will contribute to two ends simultaneously: patient-centered care and providing staff with what is required for their psychological support and motivation. Ways must be discovered, moreover, for building the means— once they have been found—into the social structure, so that they will not erode as has so often been the case after promising experiments have come to an end.

[1] Shea, Edmund J., "A Hospital Administrator Says . . . ," *Nursing Outlook*, vol. 8, March, 1960, pp. 139–140.

At present "progressive patient care" and automation in patient areas are receiving much attention.[1] They demand valuable reconsideration of environmental factors including the use of space, labor-saving machines to replace repetitive tasks that are often a source of frustration, and alterations in staffing patterns that would provide greater differentiation in patient care and perhaps greater work satisfaction. Unless very careful scrutiny is given to the psychosocial needs both of patients and staff, however, these plans are likely to revolve around degrees of sickness, procedural arrangements, and cost factors, and not significantly touch the central core of the human problem.

For that reason we wish to end the discussion by referring to a theoretical formulation of hospital reorganization that would seek to achieve dynamic equilibrium between patients and the resources of the institution, both human and nonhuman. Howard E. Wooden, its author, has now spent several years in one community hospital of about 350 beds, which he has been able to observe from "top to bottom" and where he has studied in great detail the patient care provided by some of its services. For the very reason that Mr. Wooden came to the hospital with a background in art and the humanities and had not been conditioned to its system by training, he could look at it as a social institution with fresh vision.

Persons acquainted with his articles will recall his first model of the relationships that appeared to him necessary for a patient-centered approach to hospital administration and planning for care.[2] The model was a tripod that looked like a low stool. Its seat represented patient care. The three legs represented the service resources, both human and nonhuman, labeled hospital personnel, medical staff, and facilities including equipment; they

---

[1] U. S. Public Health Service, *Elements of Progressive Patient Care*, Department of Health, Education, and Welfare, Washington, 1959; Halderman, Jack C., and Faye G. Abdellah, "Concepts of Progressive Patient Care," *Hospitals*, vol. 33, May 16, 1959, pp. 38–42, and vol. 33, June 1, 1959, pp. 41ff; Blumberg, Mark S., "Hospital Automation," *Hospitals*, vol. 35, August 1, 1961, pp. 34ff.

[2] "The Hospital's Purpose Is the Patient, But . . . ," *Modern Hospital*, vol. 92, January, 1959, pp. 9off.; and "The System May Come Ahead of the Patient," vol. 91, September, 1958, pp. 99–104. His several papers and the film now available dealing with the family-centered maternity service at St. Mary's Hospital, Evansville, Indiana, illustrate an attempt to bring patient care and the resources of the institution more nearly into dynamic equilibrium.

were regarded of equal moment as operational functions in achieving patient care. The rungs or stretchers that held the legs firmly in place portrayed the administration; its function was that of a coordinating mechanism focusing the several resources on patient needs. The tripod was shown resting firmly on a basc block identified as the community.

Obviously this model represented a major restructuring of the organizational design of the hospital. Instead of being somewhere outside the system of patterned relationships, the patient was clearly given the focal position and everything was planned to converge on meeting his requirements. Mr. Wooden later concluded, however, that this model was deficient because it was static. It ignored the impact of the roles of the various groups on one another, and lacked the capacity to accommodate change while simultaneously maintaining its state of balance. He found his second model in mobile sculpture (now familiar to almost everyone as "mobiles" used for decorative purposes) the parts of which always exist in a state of dynamic equilibrium.[1]

A mobile model of the hospital was designed and constructed, containing the same six elements appearing in the tripod. The new model, however, consists of a principal lever labeled administrative coordination, from one end of which is suspended the single leaf that designates the patient. From the other end of the lever, the three leaves symbolizing the three major resources are suspended and so arranged as to provide balance for "the patient" leaf. The entire complex is hung from an elastic net that represents the community network.

The model demonstrates that although each of the six principal parts of the system possesses separateness or individual existence, they are all nevertheless functionally interrelated, for the effect of change in one is spread to all the others. For example, a disturbance in the leaf labeled personnel, caused by some threat to the assumptions or values of the hospital staff, will be transmitted to all other parts of the organization. This model emphasizes particularly the role of administration (including supervi-

---

[1] This theoretical formulation is discussed and the mobile model of the hospital is pictured in his article, "Patient-Centered Hospital Bends in the Patient's Direction," in *Modern Hospital*, vol. 93, September, 1960, pp. 108ff.

sion) in coordinating all parts of the system in order to maintain a steady state of dynamic balance. Balance depends solely on behavioral plasticity.

The mobile system is balanced organically, for although it is a combination of diverse elements, through time and steady movement it releases its tensions by undergoing change and thereby transforms them into growth. It too is a center of conflicts but as these conflicts appear there is the appropriate adjustment so that the conflicts are resolved by an inner creative capacity. Essentially it eliminates crises within the framework of organization, not by ignoring the crises, but rather by a spontaneous on-going process of adaptation and change. Such a system thus projects an image of respect for human dignity and life needs.[1]

THE CHALLENGE OF "RESPONSIBILITY"

When Thomas Bell, the novelist, realized that time was running out for him because of inoperable cancer, he wrote a series of short essays that were published after his death under his chosen title, *In the Midst of Life*.[2] For persons working in the therapeutic milieu, these disciplined but nevertheless poignant reflections provide a resensitization to the significance of "things," of food, of the goodness of being alive—and to the reality of facing death. One of Bell's pieces of a different kind is a conversation that he carries on at five in the morning with an imaginary stranger. In the paragraphs reproduced in abbreviated form below, Bell portrays the dilemma of society everywhere, the struggle between irresponsibility and responsibility. It is this dilemma with which hospitals too are faced, and with which they must struggle if responsibility in its broader dimensions is to be "born."

The key word, I suddenly perceive, is "irresponsible." The disappearance from most people's working consciousness of a genuine sense of individual responsibility for what is going on in the world seems to me one of the really noteworthy characteristics of our time. Apparently everything has become so big and organized and bureaucratized, so *dehumanized*, that nobody feels able to influence it one way or another any more. Consequently, nobody feels responsible

[1] *Ibid.*, p. 111.
[2] Atheneum Press, New York, 1961.

when something goes wrong, whether it's a toaster that won't toast or a world war nobody wants. Who hasn't heard the universal disclaimer: Don't blame me, I just work here? Who hasn't used it?

Yet to say that nobody is responsible is only another way of saying that everybody *is*—a harsh truth if there ever was one. Every man is responsible, not only for what he himself does to his world but for what he permits others to do to it. Cain has his answer: We are all each one of us his brother's keeper whether we like it or not, whether we like him or not. It is that or extinction.

APPENDICES

Appendix 1

THE CASE OF "THE CUP CAKE TREATMENT"

by Geraldine Skinner, R.N.[1]

The setting for this story is a 2200 bed, chronic disease hospital in the Southwest of the USA. It is rather new as a hospital, but very old as an institution inasmuch as it existed for nearly seventy years as a county poor farm before it gained the title of "a chronic disease and rehabilitation general hospital." It has functioned as a custodial home for the aged since the early 1920's, and from the early 1930's until January, 1958, it cared for "mental hygiene patients." The latter program was discontinued at that time. The presence of a large mental hygiene unit in the institution had made it possible for the hospital staff to transfer certain patients from the open wards to locked wards if they did not conform to patterns of behavior that were considered desirable by medical and nursing personnel. This practice has significance for our story as the reader will see.

One fine day in 1960, Mrs. Q, head nurse on Ward X with its 42 elderly male patients, called Mrs. A, the assistant director of Nursing Service, requesting that Mr. Sam Jones, a patient on her ward, be moved to another ward. She reported that he was a stubborn old man and her attendants had put up with all they cared to from him. On the day shift Ward X was staffed with one head nurse, Mrs. Q, and four attendants, who were middle-aged women. The attendants usually worked in pairs, one on each side of the patient's bed. This resulted in a running conversation between them and a minimal amount of conversation directed to the patient.

As the result of Mrs. Q's request to have Mr. Jones transferred, a ward meeting was called. The chief supervising nurse and one of the hospital psychiatrists joined the head nurse and her attendants to confer about Mr. Jones. To initiate the conference Dr. M told the group that he understood that Sam Jones had caused them a lot of trouble. He then

[1] Director of Nursing, Rancho Los Amigos Hospital, Downey, California.

161

requested Mrs. Q and each of her attendants to explain why Sam Jones was so troublesome. Mrs. Q, who had long been a head nurse in the custodial geriatric program of this hospital, gladly spearheaded the complaint session about Mr. Jones. Each attendant followed suit, and it was learned that the patient was quite a grouch; complained frequently, did not appear to appreciate his care, and showed real hostility at times to the women attendants. He had been on this ward approximately five years, and the attendants had been working there from six months to eight years. Mrs. Q had been the head nurse for three years.

Eventually all had expressed their opinions about Sam Jones to the fullest. It would appear that their case for having him transferred elsewhere was well justified. (Since the Mental Hygiene Wards had been closed, the request for transfer meant that "someone else should care for this obstinate old man.") When the case seemed "in the bag," Dr. M inquired, "Does Sam Jones have any real friend on this ward either among staff or patients?" At this point everyone looked at each other and said, "We are good to him!" Dr. M said, "I don't mean someone who is good to him, isn't anyone a real friend to him?" There was much silence and deep thought. Dr. M continued, "Is Sam married? Is his wife living? Does he have any children? What was his occupation when well?"

After many questions and much discussion, Mrs. Q and her attendants found that they really knew very little about Mr. Jones despite the fact that they had cared for him daily for nearly five years. As their lack of information became apparent the attendants decided that they would like to learn more about him. They made up their minds that they would do so by being more friendly and using what they called "The Cup Cake Treatment." They asked the chief supervising nurse and the psychiatrist to leave him on Ward X for two more weeks while they gave the treatment. Each day one of the attendants was to have, as a special project, the Cup Cake Treatment of Sam Jones. One day he would be given a homemade cup cake, another day he would be given flowers; each day for the two-week period he would be the recipient of special attention. A second ward conference would then be scheduled.

During the ensuing two weeks the psychiatrist dropped in periodically to visit Mrs. Q to see how she and her staff were "making out" with Mr. Jones. Dr. M had a motive in stimulating the interest of this nurse who had always thought in terms of the custodial care of chronic patients rather than rehabilitation. At the time of the second ward conference the atmosphere was somewhat more exciting since all of the staff had learned a good many things about their patient. He was married, had a wife and three daughters who never came to see him despite the fact that they lived in southern California. Could this be why he disliked women in general?

It had also been discovered that his teeth had been extracted while he was being treated at another county hospital, with the result that his food was not appetizing. Gradually his hearing was failing, and he *did* need glasses. He would like to get out of bed but he had a double hernia that needed surgical attention. Everyone was surprised to learn these things. And somehow Sam hadn't been so cantankerous the past two weeks! Could Dr. M help them get him a new hearing aid? They all wanted Sam to remain on Ward X for another month.

As the reader has no doubt guessed, the staff of Ward X eventually adopted Sam Jones as their special project. He gained many friends, new glasses, a hearing aid; he was put on the list for new teeth and a bilateral hernia repair. Mrs. Q and her attendants couldn't quite understand why Sam Jones had changed so much; moreover, they were discovering that other patients on Ward X had changed too. This was a real turning point in the life of Sam Jones, just as it was also the turning point in nursing care on this unit. The attendants on Ward X have learned that geriatric care can be exciting when individualized, and that TLC is the key to much success.

Appendix 2

DETERMINATION BY THE WORK GROUP OF HOW MUCH IT WILL DO

The following brief excerpt, taken from Ira Wolfert's report of the construction of the forty-five-story Socony Mobil Building in New York City, appears on pp. 298–299 of his book, *An Epidemic of Genius*, published by Simon and Schuster, New York, 1960.

[All schedules concerning the delivery of building materials] had to be fitted into the rhythm of work of the men, who seem to have unwritten laws about how much is a good day's work. Twenty-five years ago, when there were seven waiting for the job for every one working, a bricklayer used to lay an inhumanly spectacular 700 bricks a day. Today it's 400 in New York, in St. Louis only about 250. A riveting crew does about 250 rivets a day.

But whatever rhythm the men have decided is fair for a fair dollar, they maintain. Crew members seek each other out to make up teams that go from job to job and are as proud of the quantity and quality of their work as teams of athletes. I saw a riveting crew fail one day to make its self-imposed quota. The foreman didn't speak to them, didn't have to; they were as angry at each other as a team that had lost a game.

Appendix 3

HOSPITAL HIERARCHY

by Marjorie Taubenhaus[1]

In any modern hospital a pecking order, similar to that seen in bird flocks, may be observed. Of course, differences between birds and hospitals exist. Birds determine precedence simply and quickly upon meeting. They fight. The stronger bird gains for all time the right to peck the weaker. The human beings involved in a hospital situation are accustomed to use symbols as surrogates for physical combat. These symbols are usually expressed as degrees, such as M.D., R.N., or M.Sc. However, like people, once birds have established their relative rank, a peculiar, often sonorous sound, called the threat sound, may be used to maintain superiority relationships.

There is one important point of differentiation between the bird and hospital pecking orders. It lies in the ability of the birds to recognize one another. People have had to develop elaborate systems of insignia and dress to ensure the recognition of rank that is intuitively grasped by birds. The confusing multiplicity of uniforms observed in any hospital is readily understood if we know that a three hundred to four hundred bed hospital may have about a thousand persons engaged directly or indirectly with the care of patients and the running of the hospital. Most bird flocks are not this complex. The variety of dress provides a clue to the pecking order and not a functional guide for the casual visitor to the hospital.

Top man on the hospital pecking pole is the doctor. He has invested at least eight years of his life in college and medical school for the ultimate privilege of wearing a long, loose white coat. No belt in the back, it flops freely in the breeze as the physician autocratically strides down the hospital corridors. Some lucky few in every hospital wear coats threadbare and out at the elbows; these are the chiefs of service. Brown-edged acid holes, however, denote only research workers. These

[1] Reprinted from *The Atlantic*, vol. 203, June, 1959.

command no special respect except in those obscure, rarefied circles where Nobel is more than a synonym for aristocratic.

Between the long white coat and the white-jacketed medical student (stethoscope peeping coyly from his pocket) stand the intern and resident. These wear white trousers, white jackets, and white shirts, hospital issue. This costume entitles the wearer to full respect on the wards, tolerance in the semiprivate rooms, and outraged demands for a doctor from the private suites.

Although the registered nurse may not have worked through as many schools as the doctor, she has undoubtedly worked through a great many more uniforms. She achieves the final triumph of the dress-that-stands-by-itself only after progressing through the blue of the student, doffing an apron here, and picking up a cap there. Very often black lines are added to her cap and extra pins to her dress at specified and very special milestones along the way. When she has finally graduated, with the frilly headpiece chosen by the hospital of her training (as its own announcement to the world that "This nurse does things the way we do") she is then officially qualified to say "yes" to a doctor's face and "no" behind his back to everybody else in the world. The maid, the aide, the intern in his first months of training, all must turn their cheek to her peck. They may draw small comfort from the knowledge that half the starch in her uniform probably comes from the dressing down the staff doctor has just given her.

The orderly relationships of the nursing echelons are probably the most clearly defined of any in the hospital and are reflected in a veritable rainbow array of uniforms. The trained practical nurse wears white, but without a registered nurse pin, and her consequent lack of authority to dispense medications leaves her not a social leg to stand on. The student is not only in blue and white, but for the first six months of her training she is bareheaded. Once she is capped, she is well on her way up the ladder. The nurse's aide may be in green, the orderly in tan, and who can forget the Grey Lady? Order of precedence is firmly established in these variations of color and form, and a whole organization of supervisors and directors exists to protect it.

Many large urban hospitals today have social service departments, realistically as well as self-consciously important in the framework of twentieth-century medical care. On the wards the medical social worker wears a white coat, her department identified only by a nameplate on the lapel and the oddity of the coiffure above. The social worker ranks herself ostensibly just below the physician, but in truth is answerable only to God and the psychiatrist.

The hospital chef wears white in well-respected, nonmedical tradition, but he has been outmaneuvered by the dieticians. In most restaurants and hotels all over the world the high white hat of the cook represents the acme of dictatorial prestige. But the hospital dieticians have pre-empted this authority as well as a nurse's uniform. Caught in a net of calories and low-residue diets, the chef's superiority to the green-clad dishwashers is small compensation for the pecks of the nutrition experts.

Laboratory technicians circulate through the hospital in stained white coats. At feud level with the nurses, they lack the magnificent hierarchical nursing organization. Some are experts in their own fields, highly specialized and correspondingly trained. Some are just routine test runners. But the white coat covers a multitude of skills, and the technician title gives the right to a few pecks here and there.

Some few secretaries in a hospital have fought through a right to a white coat. They are the envied ones, even though they may have to suffer the slings and arrows of outrageous surgical chiefs for their dubious privilege. For, who knows? They may one day be taken for technicians.

The nether regions, both actual and rhetorical, are inhabited by a variety of persons and uniforms. Hospitals are fond of the term "ancillary personnel," and it includes the engineers, maintenance men, and laundry workers concealed in the hospital basement as well as the maids, elevator men, and pages.

The bottom of the pecking order is represented by its own, peculiarly humiliating uniform. The hospital patient, outranked by the lowliest pantrywoman, is exposed literally and figuratively in a short white chemise. This garment, barely reaching to mid-thigh, is split the length of the back and inadequately fastened at the neck and waist with strings. If a patient thinks that his position as Chairman of the Board of twenty-two large industries gives him any status, his hospital gown is calculated to dispel the delusion.

Appendix 4

"ADD US ALL UP AND WE'RE A BUREAUCRACY"

The problem of bureaucracy or hierarchical structure is graphically described in two paragraphs of John Medelman's story, "It's Been a Long Snow," which *Harper's Magazine* published in September, 1960. A private conversation is going on between the Adjutant of the Bethel Mountain Radar Station, located in an isolated part of Alaska, and Captain Fenmer from Division Headquarters in Anchorage. The Adjutant says, "You know we don't have any of those silly power units out here. Why did you insist on my making out this report?" Captain Fenmer finally bursts out:

"It's mutual fear. . . . The whole goddam system is based on mutual fear. I was told that all units subordinate to division had to turn in those reports. I had to have a report from each unit in my file. I didn't want to invent a bunch of power units. If you wanted to, that was your business and your responsibility. I'm trying to survive. Every time Congress cuts the budget they toss out some more officers. One bad effectiveness report—that's all it takes. One guy above you who doesn't like you and you're on the first list for release. Suppose they tossed me out? Where would I go? Who'd hire me? I'm forty-three. I'm an old man on the outside."

He paused. Then he went on. "It's not very hard to survive, though. All you have to do is stay out of trouble. When you really try to do something is when you put yourself in danger. Submerge, swim along with the rest—and get it down on paper, that's the key." He leaned forward. "When you got my message, the one saying the report was mandatory, I bet you laughed. I would've once. 'What a pinhead! What a blind bureaucratic clown!' I would've said. But you've seen me. I'm no clown. You know something? I don't know any clowns in the Air Force. I work with a guy named Norman Parrish. Captain Parrish. He's no clown. He shot down four Japs in World War II. On weekends he goes off hunting rams, climbs around the mountains all by himself.

He's forty-five years old and he's tough as hell. He's a man, not a bureaucrat. And I'm a man, not a bureaucrat. But add us all up and we're a bureaucracy. It's the system. It's wrapping us all up in warm secure fat. You know something? When I sent you that 'report mandatory' message, I didn't smile cynically like you would've if you'd been sending it. Sending it seemed perfectly natural, not even worth thinking about."

Appendix 5

TRAINING FOR EFFECTIVE COMMUNICATION

The following pages have been taken, with some abbreviation, from a talk given by D. K. Waugh, Casper District Manager, The Mountain States Telephone and Telegraph Company, at the Veterans' Administration Hospital, Sheridan, Wyoming, May 23, 1958. The talk is being reproduced here with Mr. Waugh's permission for several reasons. First, it includes more valuable information, clearly summarized, than is often available in so few pages. Second, most of the material on symbols of communication, listening, and the role of the supervisor as a communication agent seems as applicable to hospitals as to the telephone company. Third, hospital and nursing administrators, who have not had an opportunity to explore the potential usefulness of training such as that provided "middle management" by some businesses and industries, will find specific reference both to content and teaching methods. Furthermore, the material itself that Mr. Waugh presents is an example of the content of the three courses he had attended and of the kind of books suggested for reading.
Preliminary to beginning the main part of his talk, Mr. Waugh described the complexity of organization of the Mountain States Telephone Company with its 26,000 employees spread over some seven states. Because of the resulting problems in communications among these employees, the "Company has from time to time instituted off-the-job training courses for supervisors at various levels."

In our discussion of communications, we have heard a great many definitions; however, of the many definitions, the one that I believe to be most clear was used by Keith Davis in his book on *Human Relations in Business*. He states that communication is "the process of passing information and understanding from one person to another." A significant point of this definition is that communications always involve two people, the sender and a receiver. One person alone cannot communicate. Only a receiver can close the communications circuit. This fact is obvious when one thinks of a man lost on an island, yelling at the top of his lungs. But it is not obvious to a manager sending out a bulletin. He tends to think that when the bulletin is sent, he has communicated.

Another significant point is that *effective* communication involves both information and understanding. A receiver may hear a sender, but still not understand what he meant. Understanding is personal in its objective, it can occur only in the receiver's mind. A supervisor may make others hear him, but he cannot make them understand him. Many supervisors overlook this fact when giving instructions or explanations. They think that telling someone is sufficient, but communication is not truly completed until that which is received is also understood. This is popularly known as "getting through" to a person.

Ten years ago, the typical supervisor in industry did not use the word "communication." He did not worry about communicating with his personnel, but times have changed. Today's leader now recognizes that communication is probably his most important responsibility. He knows that his leadership takes effect through the process of communication. If there is no communication, there is no leadership, because the leader interacts with others by communicating with them. Great leadership ideas are strictly armchair thoughts until the leader through communication puts them into effect. Communication is not an end in itself, but is the process by which ends are accomplished.

The relationship between leadership and communication is easy to understand when one thinks of a small group somewhere in a company. The group consists of a manager or supervisor and four of his men. Let us assume in the beginning, that they cannot communicate with each other. Suppose that each man has around him a complete wall made of brick and mortar, blocking all forms of communication. The wall is so high that each worker cannot even see his associates, because that would be a form of communication. It is obvious that under these conditions a supervisor cannot lead his men nor can they follow. A worker has no way of knowing what his manager wants him to do. The supervisor cannot give orders and instructions; further, he cannot motivate his people because he cannot know their needs and wants. When there is complete communication failure, the group effort is impossible.

While I have used in my illustration walls of brick and mortar, the walls that exist around persons in business are those that exist in their minds, or because they are hard to contact or difficult to understand. These barriers to communication may be just as effective as an actual physical wall. Often these human barriers are more like filter paper than a brick wall. They let through some communications, but hold back others, thereby making communication inadequate. The result is misunderstanding, lack of motivation, insecurity, conflict, and inability to make a decision. Such half-way communication gets half-way results.

If these brick and mortar walls, or "walls of silence," as we might call them, are removed from our supervisor and his men so that they can communicate, then they are able to work together. This makes it obvious that one purpose of communication is to provide the information and understanding necessary for group effort. When people can communicate, they can work together. I say that they *can* work together, but *will* they? Whether they do or not depends on their morale and attitude toward cooperation. It depends on how well the supervisor interprets their interest and the company's interests and then integrates these interests. This is another purpose of communication, to provide the attitudes necessary for motivation, cooperation, and job satisfaction. This second purpose is extremely important because there is increasing evidence that modern production problems are related more to attitudes than fundamental skills and job knowledge. These two purposes of communication can be summarized as "the skill to work" and "the will to work." The result is the joint achievement of high productivity and high job satisfaction, which makes an effective organization.

The significance of communication was illustrated early in history by the incident of the Tower of Babel. "When the Lord chose to stop the building of the tower, he confused the workers' tongues," thereby effectively ending the project. More recently, a study by the National Industrial Conference Board showed the significance of effective communication in the practical business environment.

Two plants, as nearly identical as possible, were the subject of the research. Both were represented by the same union and were located in similar towns. They were operated by the same company. The chief difference was that one of them, Plant X, had maintained an active communications program for nine years, while Plant Y had no such program.

The results were startlingly favorable to the use of a communications program. Workers' responses to the three summary questions will show how the plants differed. When the workers were asked, "Does your company do a good job of telling you what's going on and what's being planned?"—in Plant X fifty-five per cent thought it did a very good job, but only eighteen per cent in Plant Y thought so. In Plant X sixty-two per cent felt they really were a part of the company, but only twenty-nine per cent felt so in Plant Y. Forty-five per cent of Plant X considered that their company was one of the very best to work for in the community but only twenty per cent of Plant Y. For each of the three questions the company with the communications program had more than twice as many enthusiastic answers as the other company.

It is generally agreed that the communication attitude of a company tends to reflect that of its top management. If top managers establish a sound information exchange with their associates and require that the associates do likewise with others farther down the line, this spirit of information-sharing tends to cover the whole firm. A successful communication program, therefore, depends upon top management to initiate and spark it. But top management's ultimate responsibility does not relieve any other management member of his basic communication obligations. No level or area in management, no single individual, can escape this responsibility because it is inexplicably a part of the management function. Managers may delegate a small part of their communication activities to staff technicians, but the major part cannot be delegated because their leadership takes effect through communication.

A fact often overlooked is that communication is also a responsibility of every operative employee. No matter what a man's job is, he must communicate with others, sometimes more, sometimes less, and he must be able to judge when, where, and how to communicate in many instances. Communications are a responsibility of every person in an organization. The supervisor, however, is doubly responsible for communications. Like everyone else, he is responsible for communicating with others, but he also is responsible for maintenance of good communications among the personnel. When each supervisor develops good communications within his own unit, it can be joined with other units to make a chain, which will maintain good communications even in large organizations. As with chain lengths, if one understanding unit has poor communication, then those units which depend on it for communication are also weakened. If a factory superintendent fails to communicate with his foremen, they are so uninformed that their communication with workers is weakened. A strong chain of communication depends on strength in every link, which places responsibility squarely on each supervisor to maintain good communication in his unit.

COMMUNICATION SYMBOLS

Communication problems in business occur in relation to two basic frameworks. One of these is semantics, the science of meaning, and may be called the technical framework of communication. The other is organizational structure, both formal and informal, which determines the relationships of people as they communicate. Each of these frameworks I would like to discuss for a few minutes, separately.

General semantics is the science of meaning as contrasted with phonetics, the science of sounds. Communication requires that meaning be imparted from one person to another. This requirement makes communication difficult, because meaning is highly subjective. It is affected by individual differences, attitudes, experiences, and the situation at the moment. It is the essence of communication problems.

People communicate by the use of symbols which are devices that are supposed to suggest certain meanings. The communicator cannot give meaning to a receiver; instead he gives a symbol to the receiver, who then subjectively takes meaning from the symbol. This is a very personal, very human process. The meaning which the receiver takes depends on his experience and attitude, not the communicator's. If in the receiver's experience the symbol has one meaning, the communicator who insists on using the symbol with another meaning will have difficulty getting through to his receiver. Supervisors need to give major emphasis to the communication principle that transfer of meaning is aided by addressing communications in terms of the experiences and attitudes of the receivers.

Symbols can stimulate any of man's basic senses, such as hearing, seeing, and feeling, but a more practical business classification of symbols is language, pictures, and action. Supervisors live in what has been called a verbal environment. They communicate with others mostly by words and others communicate to them in the same way. The modern supervisor has difficulty doing his job unless he can use words effectively. Effective use of words does not necessarily mean proper grammar, instead it is the ability to impart to others the meaning which the supervisor intends. Language is both written and spoken. Each of these has its own particular techniques and problems.

Language has three primary functions. First, it is used to refer to that which exists or occurs in the external world outside the body of the communicator. Many of these things are subject to observation and verification. Second, language is used to express the person's attitudes, emotions, and ideas, to express the world inside himself. It is this function of language that makes it difficult to interpret what people mean. In fact, much of what people say in day-to-day interaction has different meaning apart from the immediate context of the situation in which it occurred. This is why people become so inflamed, and rightly so, when their statements are repeated out of context, or when they are held to the statements in a later different situation. The third function of language is emotional release. Many employee statements are made because of inner compulsion and feeling rather than with malicious intent. The employee is ready to forget the statement, once made, because it has served its purpose, yet management sometimes wants to "make something of it." Military organizations have long recognized this problem and they officially sanction the soldier's right to "grouse."

A second type of symbol is pictures. Business makes extensive use of pictures. It depends heavily on blueprints, charts, maps, films, three-dimensional models, and similar devices. There is an old saying to the effect that a picture can be worth a thousand words. A shoe manufacturer, who was having trouble getting his workers to maintain quality, made good use of pictures to restore careful work. He placed finished shoe rejects in a large room for several weeks and then brought representative employee groups into the room to browse around and see for themselves. Few words were spoken, but much meaning was imparted by the sight of the rejected shoes. This manager was using pictures effectively as a supplement to his language communication. Pictures are, as the term implies, visual aids, and are most effective when used with well-chosen words and actions to tell the complete story.

A third type of symbol is action. Often, managers forget that what they do is a means of communication to the extent that it is interpreted as a symbol by others. For example, a handshake and a smile have meaning. A raise in the pay envelope has meaning. Two significant points about action are often overlooked. One is that failure to act is an important form of communication. The manager has communicated when he fails to compliment someone for a job well done or fails to take a promised action. A second fact about action which managers often overlook, is that action speaks louder than words in the long run. People believe action more than they do words and pictures. The manager who says one thing but does another will find that his personnel listen most to what he does. Perhaps a short illustration would show how this works in practice.

The zone manager of a particular sales office gave considerable stress to the idea that he depended upon his men to help him do a good job because, as he stated it, "You men are the ones in direct contact with the customer, and you get lots of valuable information and useful suggestions." In most of his sales meetings he stressed the fact that he always welcomed their ideas and suggestions, but here is how he translated his words into action: in those sales meetings, the schedule was so tight that by the time he finished his pep talk, there was no time for anyone to present problems or ask questions, and he would hardly tolerate an interruption during his talk because he claimed this destroyed its punch. If a salesman tried to present a suggestion in the manager's office, the manager usually began with, "Fine, I am glad you brought in your suggestion." Before long, however, he directed the conversation to some subject in his mind or had to meet an appointment, or found some other reason for never quite getting to the suggestion. The few suggestions that did get through, he rebuffed with, "Yeah, I thought of that a long time ago, but it won't work." The eventual result was that he received no suggestions. His actions spoke louder than his words.

Of all the communication symbols, probably the two most important in employee communication are face-to-face conversation and action. They are not new, but management has a great deal to learn about how to use them for improved understanding and human relations.

Since meaning is difficult to impart, it is a natural assumption that if the symbols can be simplified, the receiver can understand them more easily. Further, if the symbols he prefers are used, he will be more receptive. This is the thinking behind the concept of readability, which seeks to make writing and speech more understandable. Readability was popularized by Rudolph Fleisch, in *The Art of Plain Talk* and *The Art of Readable Writing*. Following considerable earlier research by Fleisch and others, these men developed formulas which can be applied to house organs, bulletins, speeches, and other communications in order to determine their level of readability.

The Fleisch formula is based on a count of average sentence length and the average number of syllables for each 100 words. These two averages are applied to a scale which gives the score for reading ease. For example, an average sentence length of 15 to 17 words with 140 to 147 syllables for each 100 words rates "standard" on the Fleisch scale. Standard should be satisfactorily read and understood by an estimated eighty three per cent of adults in the United States. Research shows the unfortunate fact that only a small proportion of management literature to employees achieve standard on the scale. Bulletins, magazines, training manuals, employee handbooks, and collective bargaining contracts consistently rate "difficult" and "very difficult," which is beyond the level of satisfactory reading for the typical adult. It follows that supervisors had not applied the principle of readability, which is that a person communicates more effectively by adapting his words and style to fit the language level and ability of his receiver. Since the main purpose of communication is to be understood, supervisors should consider the receiver and try to fit his needs.

It has often been observed that the typical employee communication in business appears to be written by college people for college people. The average reader's experience has not taught him to understand such complicated writing except by carefully studying it, which he is seldom motivated to do. For example, an examination of twenty labor contracts distributed to employees showed that all rated difficult or very difficult. A study of seventy-one employee handbooks showed that sixty-five of them rated tougher than standard. Since the employees' reading levels cannot be immediately changed, perhaps those who prepare employee publications should consider their approach and make their work more readable.

As an illustration of some of the difficulties being encountered, I should like to quote from a bulletin put out by the Public Relations Department of the American Telephone and Telegraph Company.

> Keeping employees well informed has always been a major objective in the telephone business. Historically, it has been the function of the public relations department to prepare magazines, newssheets, booklets, charts, etc., to keep employees informed about the business. And we thought we were doing a pretty good job.
>
> But these surveys uncovered some weak spots. It seems that the company may pump information into an employee, overwhelm him with facts, send magazines and bulletins to his home, show him films—and all this may come to nothing. If the employee is dissatisfied with his work and his attitude is poor, the chances are that he won't go out and do an effective public relations job for the company.
>
> Getting the facts across is necessary, of course, but it is not sufficient. Let me put it this way: *Attitude* is the key to whether an employee tries to do a job in the company's behalf; *facts* help him succeed, once his attitude is favorable.
>
> Again, in the course of these surveys, employees had a great deal to say also about the *content* of our informational activities. From these comments, we concluded:
>
> 1. Very often, company communications to employees fail to reach them, let alone get passed on by them to others, because the information is not actually absorbed or understood.
>
> 2. Much of what is communicated lacks interest or personal reference for employees.
>
> 3. Some employees feel that we give them too many facts at once; they can't remember all they are told even if they try to.
>
> 4. Some kinds of factual information seem to have only a limited employee audience.

These findings refer to weaknesses in our formal or printed communications rather than in regular day-to-day communication between employee and supervisor. In our formal communications, do we tend to emphasize what we, as management, believe employees ought to know rather than what they want to know? Perhaps we should listen more closely to employees and discover what kinds of information they need. As some employees have observed: "If the company wants us to be interested in its problems, then the company should be interested in our problems."

To take this a bit farther, here is what employees tell us about the ways in which we communicate with them:

1. Small, two-way meetings are most effective if (a) the atmosphere is such as to encourage free discussion and upward communication; and (b) groups are small and informal (six to ten people).

2. The supervisor's role as communicator varies tremendously, depending on such things as: (a) his own personality and how well trained he is as a communicator; (b) his relations, in other connections, with the employees to whom he is communicating; (c) whether he is accepted by employees as an authority on the subject under discussion; and (d) how much he believes in what he is asked to do. (The role of the supervisor appears to be of first importance. In other research, employees told us they were getting most of their information about the company from printed matter, but would prefer to get it from their supervisors.)

3. Movies seem to have greater impact than printed matter; they are most valuable, however, when followed by discussion.

4. Written materials—unless they have at least local or, ideally, personal references—are the least effective means of communicating information to employees. There is almost universal resistance to reading bare facts and figures.

LISTENING

If meaning is to be imparted in communication, then the concept of listening assumes special importance. The reason for its significance becomes evident by reference to the well-known sport of tennis. A tennis player, if he serves the ball cannot then say to himself, "My shot will be an overhead volley into the back court." His next shot has to depend on how his opponent returns the ball. He may have an overall strategy, but each of his shots must be conditioned by how the ball is returned. Unless he does condition his shots, he will soon find himself swinging aimlessly and losing a game.

Every speaker and listener needs to realize that spoken communication has a back and forth pattern, similar to the exchange of play between tennis players. The speakers send symbols and receivers' responses come back to the speaker. The result is a developing play-by-play situation in which the speaker can adjust his message to fit the responses of his receiver. This opportunity to adjust to the receiver is the one great advantage of speaking compared to writing, but the advantage is lost if the speaker does not listen, and the message is lost if the intended listener does not listen. Listening is, therefore, important to both parties in conversational interchange. Listening is a dual responsibility of speaker and listener. The major benefits of good listening are:

1. A good listener can make better decisions because he has better information.
2. A good listener saves time because he learns more within a given period of time.
3. Listening helps the communicator to determine how well his message is being received.
4. A good listener stimulates others to better speaking.
5. Good listening decreases misunderstanding.

Listening consumes a large part of most supervisors' jobs. Research shows that the typical supervisor spends thirty-five to fifty-five per cent of his time listening, yet the average listener two months later remembers only about twenty-five per cent of what was said. Even immediately after listening, tests indicate that listeners have missed significant parts of the communications; therefore, there is a real need for improving listening in business. Fortunately, nearly any person can improve his listening. Experience suggests that proper training and practice can increase listening comprehension by at least twenty-five per cent, usually much more.

It is essential that the listener approach the situation with a positive attitude and a desire to listen. He must keep his mind open, regardless of what statements are made or appear to be forthcoming. Since the average person speaks about 125 words per minute, the listener's thought processes run from three to five times as fast. Listeners need to concentrate forcefully on the message in order to keep from daydreaming or mind-wandering to another subject. Listening is a conscious, positive act, requiring will power. It is not a simple passive exposure to sound. Each listener's job is to listen to ideas rather than to each individual word of the speaker. As we know, most words have several meanings, and listening only to words raises questions and confuses the listener. Listening to words is often quite apparent with children when they, in their uninhibited manner, interrupt the speaker to ask about a word before he finishes his sentence. Listeners should look to the meaning, not the words.

Let us examine for a few minutes the informal communication system, or "grapevine" as it is more commonly known. Most managers prefer to use only formal communication because they can control it, but they must also deal with the grapevine. Grapevine is ordinarily considered undesirable and attempts have been made to abolish it. However, it can be good.

1. It gives the supervisor insight into employee attitudes.
2. Is a safety valve for employee emotions.
3. Helps spread useful information by interpreting management's formal orders into the language of the workers so that it is more easily understood.

Undesirable qualities:

1. It spreads rumor and untruth, since it is sometimes built on a "grain of truth," regarding lay-off, transfer, dismissal, etc.
2. Travels at a fast pace. As an example, during recent bargaining sessions it was necessary for the public relations department to work all night getting out a bulletin on the settlement reached, in order to beat the grapevine and be sure employees had the correct information promptly.

The grapevine is influential. Managers are beginning to realize that they need to learn its habits and seek to guide it. They should observe these points:

Listen to it.
Learn who the principal leaders are.
Learn how it operates.
Learn what information it carries.
Realize that it is sometimes necessary to attack untruths or misinformation.
Combat them by use of a coffee-break column, bulletins, news releases, etc.

SHORT TRAINING COURSES FOR SUPERVISORS

Earlier, I spoke of formal training used by our company and other Bell System companies in the training of supervisors for more effective communication. One of the first courses consisted of two weeks, off-the-job training in principles of human relations, during which the following items that stressed positive action were studied:

Perfect self-control.
Appreciate and praise.
Stress rewards, avoid punishment.
Criticize tactfully.
Always listen.
Explain thoroughly.
Consider your men's interests as you would your own.

Another interesting course given to our supervisors, which I believe has helped the participants a great deal, was entitled "Talking with People." In this course, the following principles were stressed:

Learn to listen.
Put others at ease by pleasing manner.
Use listening responses.
Encourage talk by lead-off questions and the use of listening responses.
Follow up key thoughts by the use of open questions, using What, When, Who, How, Where, and Which. Such questions cannot be answered by a Yes or No.
And again, use listening responses.

A listening response is a short comment or act made to another person to convey the idea that you are interested, attentive, and wish him to continue. It is made quietly and briefly, usually when the speaker pauses, so as not to interfere with his train of thought.
There are five types of listening responses:

1. Nod	Nodding the head slightly and waiting.
2. Pause	Looking at the speaker expectantly without doing or saying anything.
3. Casual Remark	"I see," "Uh-huh," "Is that so," "That's interesting," etc.
4. Echo	Repeating the last few words the speaker said.
5. Mirror	Reflecting back to the speaker your understanding of what he has just said. (You feel that ————)

Another course which was both interesting and useful was known as "Coaching." In the Mountain States Telephone Company, as in many other organizations, considerable emphasis is being placed on the coaching function of supervisors on the higher levels.

There are seven things a boss needs to do if he is to succeed as a coach or developer of management talent:

> He must establish and maintain a climate that encourages and stimulates growth.
> Guide his subordinates, drawing on his own experiences.
> Counsel them, giving sound advice—but only when needed.
> Encourage them and demonstrate by example the use of basic management skills and procedures.
> Give them special assignments and arrange for cross-training when he feels it will fill a definite need.
> Stimulate development by supplying proper incentives.
> Challenge them by delegating a full measure of authority, thus forcing practice in decision-making.

Coaching points up the responsibility which managers have in developing persons who work under them. Training off the job, special schools and courses—all these are useful in the total development approach. But ultimately, progress and skill improvement of any man is the primary responsibility of the man himself and of his boss, and cannot be evaded by either.

In all of the courses, a certain amount of role-playing was used in an attempt to have each person get the feel of attitudes and reactions in the various roles. For instance, a person at one time might be playing the role of the supervisor, and immediately afterward be playing the role of the employee opposite the supervisor in the same situation. I have a niece who is a teacher of second-grade pupils. In discussing a course with her one day, I mentioned that we used role-playing extensively in it. She stated that she found role-playing effective in the second grade, also. Her students were constantly playing roles of one kind or another in portraying various stories. As I think back over the years of schooling, I believe that role-playing has been an important part of the process of instruction.

Appendix 6

HOW A NURSING SERVICE CREATES AND USES THE SOCIAL SYSTEM TO PROTECT ITSELF AGAINST ANXIETY

The excerpt presented below has been taken from pages 101–109 of Isabel E. P. Menzies' "A Case-Study in the Functioning of Social Systems as a Defence Against Anxiety: A Report of a Study of the Nursing Service of a General Hospital," published in *Human Relations*, vol. 13, no. 2, 1960. The London "hospital" studied consisted of a general hospital with 500 beds, outpatient services, and a nurse-training school; three small specialist hospitals; and a convalescent home. This group of institutions had an integrated nursing service run by a matron located in the main hospital. The nursing staff and students were used interchangeably among the four units. The total nursing personnel numbered about 700, of whom 150 were graduate nurses and the rest were students. The graduate nurses were employed in administrative, supervisory, and teaching roles; the students provided the staff nursing, except for some direct patient care given by graduate nurses who were on the patient floors in a supervisory or teaching capacity.

Interviews with nurses individually and in small groups, observation of operational units, and informal contacts pointed to a high level of tension, distress, and anxiety within the nursing service. Miss Menzies "found it hard to understand how nurses could tolerate so much anxiety." Certain facts seemed to indicate that they could not: the withdrawal before graduation of one-third of the students, the frequent changing of positions by the graduate nurses, and the high sickness rates for minor illnesses.

It was Miss Menzies' conclusion, as a psychoanalyst, that patient care is so anxiety-inducing for nurses (who "bear the full, immediate, and concentrated impact of stresses" arising from it) that over a long period of time the nursing service has, often unconsciously, developed a particular kind of social system. This system is designed to protect the individual nurse against anxiety, guilt, doubt, and uncertainty. Little attempt has been made positively to help her confront anxiety-evoking experiences. As a result, although anxiety is to some extent contained, "true mastery of anxiety by deep working-through and modification is seriously inhibited. Thus it is to be expected that nurses will persistently experience a higher degree of anxiety than is justified by the objective situation alone." The very social system, moreover, that evolved as a defense against anxiety fosters frustration and deprives nurses of greatly needed reassurance and satisfactions.

In the pages from her study reprinted here, Miss Menzies describes specific defensive techniques associated with the social system that the nursing service uses in this struggle against anxiety; she does not consider how physicians and patients may also be used for the same purpose. Although there are various differences between the social system of the group of hospitals described and hospitals in the United States, most of the "defenses" will appear familiar to the reader. It must be kept in mind that Miss Menzies' interpretation of the social system is a psychoanalytical one. Persons trained in other theoretical frames of reference, such as sociologists, would interpret the social system somewhat differently. This particular analysis is so thought-provoking, however, that it deserves careful consideration.

Splitting Up the Nurse-Patient Relationship. The core of the anxiety situation for the nurse lies in her relation with the patient. The closer and more concentrated this relationship, the more the nurse is likely to experience the impact of anxiety. The nursing service attempts to protect her from the anxiety by splitting up her contact with patients. It is hardly too much to say that the nurse does not nurse patients. The total work-load of a ward or department is broken down into lists of tasks, each of which is allocated to a particular nurse. She performs her patient-centred tasks for a large number of patients, perhaps as many as all the patients in the ward, often 30 or more in number. As a corollary, she performs only a few tasks for, and has restricted contact with, any one patient. This prevents her from coming effectively into contact with the totality of any one patient and his illness and offers some protection from the anxiety this arouses.

Depersonalization, Categorization, and Denial of the Significance of the Individual. The protection afforded by the task-list system is reinforced by a number of other devices that inhibit the development of a full person-to-person relationship between nurse and patient, with its consequent anxiety. The implicit aim of such devices, which operate both structurally and culturally, may be described as a kind of depersonalization or elimination of individual distinctiveness in both nurse and patient. For example, nurses often talk about patients, not by name, but by bed numbers or by their diseases or a diseased organ, "the liver in bed 10" or "the pneumonia in bed 15." Nurses themselves deprecate this practice, but it persists. Nor should one underestimate the difficulties of remembering the names of say 30 patients on a ward, especially the high-turnover wards. There is an almost explicit "ethic" that any patient must be the same as any other patient. It must not matter to the nurse whom she nurses or what illness. Nurses find it extraordinarily difficult to express preferences even for types of patients or for men or women patients. If pressed to do so, they tend to add rather guiltily some remark like "You can't help it." Conversely, it should not matter to the patient which nurse attends him or, indeed, how many different nurses do. By implication it is the duty as well as the need and privilege of the patient to be nursed and of the nurse to nurse, regardless of the fact that a patient may greatly need to "nurse" a distressed nurse and nurses may sometimes need to be "nursed." Outside the specific requirements of his physical illness and treatment, the way a patient is nursed is determined largely by his membership in the category patient and minimally by his idiosyncratic wants and needs. For example, there is one way only of bed-making, except when the physical illness requires another; only one time to wash all patients in the morning.

The nurses' uniforms are a symbol of an expected inner and behavioural uniformity; a nurse becomes a kind of agglomeration of nursing skills, without individuality; each is thus perfectly interchangeable with another of the same skill-level. Socially permitted differences between nurses tend to be restricted to a few major categories, outwardly differentiated by minor differences in insignia on the same basic uniform, an arm stripe for a second-year nurse, a slightly different cap for a third-year nurse. This attempts to create an operational identity between all nurses in the same category. To an extent indicating clearly the need for "blanket" decisions, duties and privileges are accorded to categories of people and not to individuals according to their personal capacities and needs. This also helps to eliminate painful and difficult decisions, e.g. about which duties and privileges should fall to each individual. Something of the same reduction of individual distinctiveness exists between operational sub-units. Attempts are made to standardize all equipment and layout to the limits allowed by their different nursing tasks, but disregarding the idiosyncratic social and psychological resources and needs of each unit.

Detachment and Denial of Feelings. A necessary psychological task for the entrant into any profession that works with people is the development of adequate professional detachment. He must learn, for example, to control his feelings, refrain from excessive involvement, avoid disturbing identifications, maintain his professional independence against manipulation and demands for unprofessional behaviour. To some extent the reduction of individual distinctiveness aids detachment by minimizing the mutual interaction of personalities, which might lead to "attachment." It is reinforced by an implicit operational policy of "detachment." "A good nurse doesn't mind moving." A "good nurse" is willing and able without disturbance to move from ward to ward or even hospital to hospital at a moment's notice. Such moves are frequent and often sudden, particularly for student nurses. The implicit rationale appears to be that a student nurse will learn to be detached psychologically if she has sufficient experience in being detached literally and physically. Most senior nurses do not subscribe personally to this implicit rationale. They are aware of the personal distress as well as the operational disturbance caused by over-frequent moves. Indeed this was a major factor in the decision to initiate our study. However, in their formal roles in the hierarchy they continue to initiate frequent moves and make little other training provision for developing genuine professional detachment. The pain and distress of breaking relationships and the importance of stable and continuing relationships are implicitly denied by the system, although they are often stressed personally, i.e. non-professionally, by people in the system.

This implicit denial is reinforced by the denial of the disturbing feelings that arise within relationships. Interpersonal repressive techniques are culturally required and typically used to deal with emotional stress. Both student nurses and staff show panic about emotional outbursts. Brisk, reassuring behaviour and advice of the "stiff upper lip," "pull yourself together" variety are characteristic. Student nurses suffer most severely from emotional strain and habitually complain that the senior staff do not understand and make no effort to help them. Indeed, when the emotional stress arises from the nurse's having made a mistake, she is usually reprimanded instead of being helped. A student nurse told me that she had made a mistake that hastened the death of a dying patient. She was reprimanded separately by four senior nurses. Only the headmistress of her former school tried to help her as a person who was severely distressed, guilty, and frightened. However, students are wrong when they say that senior nurses do not understand or feel for their distress. In personal conversation with us, seniors showed considerable understanding and sympathy and often remembered surprisingly vividly some of the agonies of their own training. But they lacked confidence in their ability to handle emotional stress in any way other than by repressive techniques, and often said, "In any case, the students won't come and talk to us." Kindly, sympathetic handling of emotional stress between staff and student nurses is, in any case, inconsistent with traditional nursing roles and relationships, which require repression, discipline, and reprimand from senior to junior.

The Attempt to Eliminate Decisions by Ritual Task-Performance. Making a decision implies making a choice between different possible courses of action and committing oneself to one of them; the choice being made in the absence of full factual information about the effects of the choice. If the facts were fully known, no decision need be made; the proper course of action would be self-evident. All decisions are thus necessarily attended by some uncertainty about their outcome and consequently by some conflict and anxiety, which will last until the outcome is known. The anxiety consequent on decision-making is likely to be acute if a decision affects the treatment and welfare of patients. To spare staff this anxiety, the nursing service attempts to minimize the number and variety of decisions that must be made. For example, the student nurse is instructed to perform her task-list in a way reminiscent of performing a ritual. Precise instructions are given about the way each task must be performed, the order of the tasks, and the time for their performance, although such precise instructions are not objectively necessary, or even wholly desirable.

If several efficient methods of performing a task exist, e.g. for bed-making or lifting a patient, one is selected and exclusively used. Much time and effort are expended in standardizing nursing procedures in cases where there are a number of effective alternatives. Both teachers and practical-work supervisors impress on the student nurse from the beginning of her training the importance of carrying out the "ritual." They reinforce this by fostering an attitude to work that regards every task as almost a matter of life and death, to be treated with appropriate seriousness. This applies even to those tasks that could be effectively performed by an unskilled lay person. As a corollary, the student nurse is actively discouraged from using her own discretion and initiative to plan her work realistically in relation to the objective situation, e.g. at times of crisis to discriminate between tasks on the grounds of urgency or relative importance and to act accordingly. Student nurses are the "staff" most affected by "rituals," since ritualization is easy to apply to their roles and tasks, but attempts are also made to ritualize the task-structure of the more complex senior staff roles and to standardize the task-performance.

Reducing the Weight of Responsibility in Decision-Making by Checks and Counter-Checks. The psychological burden of anxiety arising from a final, committing decision by a single person is dissipated in a number of ways, so that its impact is reduced. The final act of commitment is postponed by a common practice of checking and re-checking decisions for validity and postponing action as long as possible. Executive action following decisions is also checked and re-checked habitually at intervening stages. Individuals spend much time in private rumination over decisions and actions. Whenever possible, they involve other nurses in decision-making and in reviewing actions. The nursing procedures prescribe considerable checking between individuals, but it is also a strongly developed habit among nurses outside areas of prescribed behaviour. The practice of checking and counter-checking is applied not only to situations where mistakes may have serious consequences, such as in giving dangerous drugs, but to many situations where the implications of a decision are of only the slightest consequence, e.g. on one occasion a decision about which of several rooms, all equally available, should be used for a research interview. Nurses consult not only their immediate seniors but also their juniors and nurses or other staff with whom they have no functional relationship but who just happen to be available.

Collusive Social Redistribution of Responsibility and Irresponsibility. Each nurse must face and, in some way, resolve a painful conflict over accepting the responsibilities of her role. The nursing task tends to evoke a strong sense of responsibility in nurses, and nurses often discharge their duties at considerable personal cost. On the other hand, the heavy burden of responsibility is difficult to bear consistently, and nurses are tempted to give it up. In addition, each nurse has wishes and impulses that would lead to irresponsible action, e.g. to scamp boring, repetitive tasks or to become libidinally or emotionally attached to patients. The balance of opposing forces in the conflict varies between individuals, i.e. some are naturally "more responsible" than others, but the conflict is always present. To experience this conflict fully and intrapsychically would be extremely stressful. The intrapsychic conflict is alleviated, at least as far as the conscious experiences of nurses are concerned, by a technique that partly converts it into an interpersonal conflict. People in certain roles tend to be described as "responsible" by themselves and to some extent by others, and in other roles people are described as "irresponsible." Nurses habitually complain that other nurses are irresponsible, behave carelessly and impulsively, and in consequence must be ceaselessly supervised and disciplined. The complaints commonly refer not to individuals or to specific incidents but to whole categories of nurses, usually a category junior to the speaker. The implication is that the juniors are not only less responsible now than the speaker, but also less responsible than she was when she was in the same junior position. Few nurses recognize or admit such tendencies. Only the most junior nurses are likely to admit these tendencies in themselves and then justify them on the grounds that everybody treats them as though they were irresponsible. On the other hand, many people complain that their seniors as a category impose unnecessarily strict and repressive discipline, and treat them as though they have no sense of responsibility. Few senior staff seem able to recognize such features in their own behaviour to subordinates. Those "juniors" and "seniors" are, with few exceptions, the same people viewed from above or below, as the case may be.

We came to realize that the complaints stem from a collusive system of denial, splitting, and projection that is culturally acceptable to, indeed culturally required of, nurses. Each nurse tends to split off aspects of herself from her conscious personality and to project them into other nurses. Her irresponsible impulses, which she fears she cannot control, are attributed to her juniors. Her painfully severe attitude to these impulses and burdensome sense of responsibility are attributed to her seniors. Consequently, she identifies juniors with her irresponsible self and treats them with the severity that self is felt to deserve. Similarly, she identifies seniors with her own harsh disciplinary attitude to her irresponsible self and expects harsh discipline. There is psychic truth in the assertion that juniors are irresponsible and seniors harsh disciplinarians. These are the roles assigned to them. There is also objective truth, since people act objectively on the psychic roles assigned to them. Discipline is often harsh and sometimes unfair, since the multiple projection also leads the senior to identify all juniors with her irresponsible self and so with each other. Thus, she fails to discriminate between them sufficiently. Nurses complain about being reprimanded for other people's mistakes while no serious effort is made to find the real culprit. A staff nurse said, "If a mistake has been made, you must reprimand someone, even if you don't know who really did it." Irresponsible behaviour was also quite common, mainly in tasks remote from direct patient-care. The interpersonal conflict is painful, as the complaints show, but is less so than experiencing the conflict fully intrapsychically, and it can more easily be evaded. The disciplining eye of seniors cannot follow juniors all the time, nor does the junior confront her senior with irresponsibility all the time.

Purposeful Obscurity in the Formal Distribution of Responsibility. Additional protection from the impact of specific responsibility for specific tasks is given by the fact that the formal structure and role system fail to define fully enough who is responsible for what and to whom. This matches and objectifies the obscurity about the location of psychic responsibility that inevitably arises from the massive system of projection described above. The content of roles and the boundaries of roles are very obscure, especially at senior levels. The responsibilities are more onerous at this level so that protection is felt as very necessary. Also the more complex roles and role-relationships make it easier to evade definition. As described above, the content of the role of the student nurse is rigidly prescribed by her task-list. However, in practice, she is unlikely to have the same task-list for any length of time. She may, and frequently does, have two completely different task-lists in a single day. There is therefore a lack of stable person-role constellations, and it becomes very difficult to assign responsibility finally to a person, a role, or a person-role constellation. We experienced this obscurity frequently in our work in the hospital, finding great difficulty, for example, in learning who should make arrangements or give permission for nurses to participate in various research activities.

Responsibility and authority on wards are generalized in a way that makes them non-specific and prevents them from falling firmly on one person, even the sister. Each nurse is held to be responsible for the work of every nurse junior to her. Junior, in this context, implies no hierarchical relationship, and is determined only by the length of time a student nurse has been in training, and all students are "junior" to trained staff. A student nurse in the fourth quarter of her fourth year is by implication responsible for all other student nurses on the ward; a student nurse in the third quarter of her fourth year for all student nurses except the previous one, and so on. Every nurse is expected to initiate disciplinary action in relation to any failure by any junior nurse. Such diffused responsibility means, of course, that responsibility is not generally experienced specifically or seriously.

The Reduction of the Impact of Responsibility by Delegation to Superiors. The ordinary usage of the word "delegation" in relation to tasks implies that a superior hands over a task and the direct responsibility for its detailed performance to subordinates, while he retains a general, supervisory responsibility. In the hospital, almost the opposite seems to happen frequently, i.e. tasks are frequently forced upwards in the hierarchy, so that all responsibility for their performance can be disclaimed. In so far as this happens, the heavy burden of responsibility on the individual is reduced.

The results of many years of this practice are visible in the nursing service. We were struck repeatedly by the low level of tasks carried out by nursing staff and students in relation to their personal ability, skill, and position in the hierarchy. Formally and informally, tasks are assigned to staff at a level well above that at which one finds comparable tasks in other institutions, while the tasks are organized so as effectively to prevent their delegation to an appropriate lower level, e.g. by clarifying policy. The task of allocating student nurses to practical duties was a case in point. The detailed work of allocating student nurses was carried out by the first and second assistant matrons and took up a considerable proportion of their working-time. In our opinion, the task is, in fact, such that, if policy were clearly defined and the task appropriately organized, it could be efficiently performed by a competent clerk part-time under the supervision of a senior nurse, who need spend little time on it. We were able to watch this "delegation upwards" in operation a number of times as new tasks developed for nurses out of changes resulting from our study. For example, the senior staff decided to change the practical training for fourth-year nurses so that they might have better training than formerly in administration and supervision. This implied, among other things, that they should spend six months continuously in one operational unit during which time they would act as understudy-cum-shadow to the sister or the staff nurse. In the circumstances, personal compatibility was felt to be very important, and it was suggested that the sisters should take part in the selection of the fourth-year students for their own wards. At first, there was enthusiasm for the proposal, but as definite plans were made and the intermediate staff began to feel that they had no developed skill for selection, they requested that, after all, senior staff should continue to select for them as they had always done. The senior staff, although already overburdened, willingly accepted the task.

The repeated occurrence of such incidents by mutual collusive agreement between superiors and subordinates is hardly surprising considering the mutual projection system described above. Nurses as subordinates tend to feel very dependent on their superiors in whom they psychically vest by projection some of the best and most competent parts of themselves. They feel that their projections give them the right to expect their superiors to undertake their tasks and make decisions for them. On the other hand, nurses, as superiors, do not feel they can fully trust their subordinates in whom they psychically vest the irresponsible and incompetent parts of themselves. Their acceptance of their subordinates' projections also conveys a sense of duty to accept their subordinates' responsibilities.

Idealization and Underestimation of Personal Development Possibilities. In order to reduce anxiety about the continuous efficient performance of nursing tasks, nurses seek assurance that the nursing service is staffed with responsible, competent people. To a considerable extent, the hospital deals with this problem by an attempt to recruit and select "staff," i.e. student nurses, who are already highly mature and responsible people. This is reflected in phrases like "nurses are born not made" or "nursing is a vocation." This amounts to a kind of idealization of the potential nursing recruit, and implies a belief that responsibility and personal maturity cannot be "taught" or even greatly developed. As a corollary, the training system is mainly orientated to the communication of essential facts and techniques, and pays minimal attention to teaching events oriented to personal maturation within the professional setting. There is no individual supervision of student nurses, and no small group teaching event concerned specifically to help student nurses work over the impact of their first essays in nursing practice and handle more effectively their relations with patients and their own emotional reactions. The nursing service must face the dilemma that, while a strong sense of responsibility and discipline are felt to be necessary for the welfare of patients, a considerable proportion of actual nursing tasks are extremely simple. This hospital, in common with most similar British hospitals, has attempted to solve this dilemma by the recruitment of large numbers of high-level student nurses who, it is hoped, are prepared to accept the temporary lowering of their operational level because they are in training.

This throws new light on the problem of the 30 per cent to 50 per cent wastage of student nurses in this and other British hospitals. It has long been treated as a serious problem and much effort has been expended on trying to solve it. In fact, it can be seen as an *essential* element in the social defence system. The need for responsible semi-skilled staff greatly exceeds the need for fully trained staff, e.g. by almost four to one in this hospital. If large numbers of student nurses do *not* fail to finish their training, the nursing profession risks being flooded with trained staff for whom there are no jobs. The wastage is, therefore, an unconscious device to maintain the balance between staff of different levels of skill while all are at a high personal level. It is understandable that apparently determined efforts to reduce wastage have so far failed, except in one or two hospitals.

Avoidance of Change. Change is inevitably to some extent an excursion into the unknown. It implies a commitment to future events that are not entirely predictable and to their consequences, and inevitably provokes doubt and anxiety. Any significant change within a social system implies changes in existing social relationships and in social structure. It follows that any significant social change implies a change in the operation of the social system as a defence system. While this change is proceeding, i.e. while social defences are being re-structured, anxiety is likely to be more open and intense. E. Jaques ["Social Systems as a Defense against Persecutory and Depressive Anxiety" in *New Directions in Psychoanalysis*, Basic Books, New York, 1955] has stressed that resistance to social change can be better understood if it is seen as the resistance of groups of people unconsciously clinging to existing institutions because changes threaten existing social defences against deep and intense anxieties.

It is understandable that the nursing service, whose tasks stimulate such primitive and intense anxieties, should anticipate change with unusually severe anxiety. In order to avoid this anxiety, the service tries to avoid change wherever possible, almost, one might say, at all cost, and tends to cling to the familiar even when the familiar has obviously ceased to be appropriate or relevant. Changes tend to be initiated only at the point of crisis. The presenting problem was a good example of this difficulty in initiating and carrying through change. Staff and student nurses had for long felt that the methods in operation were unsatisfactory and had wanted to change them. They had, however, been unable to do so. The anxieties and uncertainties about possible changes and their consequences inhibited constructive and realistic planning and decision. At least, the present difficulties were familiar and they had some ability to handle them. The problem was approaching the point of breakdown and the limits of the capacities of the people concerned when we were called in. Many other examples of this clinging to the inappropriate familiar could be observed. For example, changes in medical practice and the initiation of the National Health Service have led to more rapid patient turnover, an increase in the proportion of acutely ill patients, a wider range of illness to be nursed in each ward, and greater variation in the work-load of a ward from day to day. These changes all point to the need for increasing flexibility in the work organization of nurses in wards. In fact, no such increase in flexibility has taken place in this hospital. Indeed, the difficulty inherent in trying to deal with a fluctuating work-load by the rather rigid system described above has tended to be handled by increased prescription and rigidity and by reiteration of the familiar. As far as one could gather, the greater the anxiety the greater the need for such reassurance in rather compulsive repetition.

The changing demands on nurses described above necessitate a growing amount of increasingly technically skilled nursing care. This has not, however, led to any examination of the implicit policy that nursing can be carried out largely by semi-qualified student nurses.